You needed it then...you need it now... you'll need it tomorrow.

Get the drug facts every nurse ne

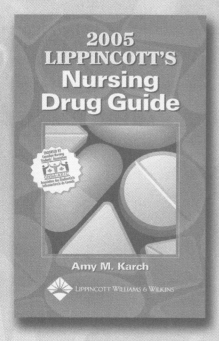
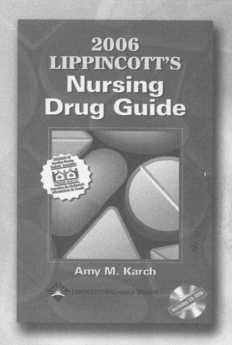
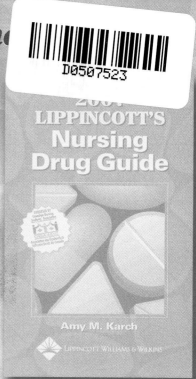

Lippincott's Nursing Drug Guide

Amy M. Karch, RN, MS

Assistant Clinical Professor, University of Rochester School of Nursing, Rochester, NY

Endorsed by the Canadian Nursing Student Association, the **Lippincott's Nursing Drug Guide** provides quick A-to-Z access to current, vital drug information.

Featuring Canadian brand names of drugs, a Canadian Regulations appendix, as well as other helpful features, the **Lippincott's Nursing Drug Guide** is the book geared for you!

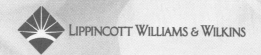
LIPPINCOTT WILLIAMS & WILKINS

Available at your local health science bookstore

If you are a faculty member interested in reviewing a copy for adoption purposes, please contact your Lippincott Williams & Wilkins sales representative at 800-399-3110.

A5G246F

A Nurse's Guide to

Dosage Calculation

Giving Medications Safely

A Nurse's Guide to
Dosage
Calculation

Giving Medications Safely

Vicki Niblett, RN, BScN

Professor/Academic Coordinator
Brock University/Loyalist College
Collaborative Nursing Baccalaureate Program
Loyalist College of Applied Arts and Technology
Belleville, Ontario, Canada

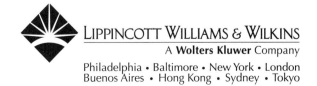

LIPPINCOTT WILLIAMS & WILKINS
A **Wolters Kluwer** Company
Philadelphia • Baltimore • New York • London
Buenos Aires • Hong Kong • Sydney • Tokyo

Senior Acquisitions Editor: Margaret Zuccarini
Managing Editor: Michelle Clarke
Editorial Assistant: Delema Caldwell-Jordan
Production Project Manager: Cynthia Rudy
Director of Nursing Production: Helen Ewan
Senior Managing Editor / Production: Erika Kors
Art Director: Joan Wendt
Manufacturing Coordinator: Karin Duffield
Production Services / Compositor: Schawk, Inc.
Printer: Courier–Kendallville

9 8 7 6 5 4 3 2 1

Library of Congress Cataloging-in-Publication Data

Niblett, Vicki.
    A nurse's guide to dosage calculation : giving medications safely / Vicki Niblett.
       p. ; cm.
    Includes index.
    ISBN 0-7817-5853-X (alk. paper)
    1. Pharmaceutical arithmetic. 2. Nursing—Mathematics. I. Title.
    [DNLM: 1. Pharmaceutical Preparations—administration & dosage—Nurses'
Instruction. 2. Drug Administration Routes—Nurses' Instruction. QV 748 N579n 2006]
RS57.N57 2006
615'.14'01513—dc22
                                                                                2005021822

Care has been taken to confirm the accuracy of the information presented and to describe generally accepted practices. However, the author, editors, and publisher are not responsible for errors or omissions or for any consequences from application of the information in this book and make no warranty, express or implied, with respect to the content of the publication.

The author, editors, and publisher have exerted every effort to ensure that drug selection and dosage set forth in this text are in accordance with the current recommendations and practice at the time of publication. However, in view of ongoing research, changes in government regulations, and the constant flow of information relating to drug therapy and drug reactions, the reader is urged to check the package insert for each drug for any change in indications and dosage and for added warnings and precautions. This is particularly important when the recommended agent is a new or infrequently employed drug.

Some drugs and medical devices presented in this publication have Food and Drug Administration (FDA) clearance for limited use in restricted research settings. It is the responsibility of the health care provider to ascertain the FDA status of each drug or device planned for use in his or her clinical practice.

LWW.com

Reviewers

Diana J. Adams, RN, MHA
Clinical Instructor
Ryerson University
Toronto, Ontario

Larisa Aponiuk, RN
Nursing Professor
Cambrian College of Applied Arts & Technology
Sudbury, Ontario

Virginia Birnie
Nurse Educator
Camosun College
Victoria, British Columbia

Hope Graham, MN, BScN, RN
Assistant Professor
St. Francis Xavier University
Antigonish, Nova Scotia

Melanie S. Macneil, RN, BScN, MSN, PhD
Assistant Professor
Brock University
St. Catharines, Ontario

Christy Raymond, RN, BScN, MEd
Coordinator/Faculty
Grant MacEwan College School of Nursing
Edmonton, Alberta

Kathleen Stevens, RN, MN
Instructional Resource Centre Coordinator
Centre for Nursing Studies
St. John's, Newfoundland

Nancy A. Walton, RN, BScN, PhD
Associate Professor
Ryerson University
Toronto, Ontario

Karen S. Webber, MN, RN
Associate Professor
Memorial University of Newfoundland
School of Nursing
St. John's, Newfoundland

Preface

Nurses play a major role in the management of health care. For those of us who work in institutional settings, one of our critical roles is administering medications safely. Safe practice includes the traditional five "rights" of medication administration—right patient, right drug, right dose, right time, and right route. Some of us include a sixth right—right documentation.

In more than 20 years of teaching nursing and supervising clinical practice, I have spent a large proportion of my time helping students work their way through the intricacies of administering medications. As well as helping them learn to carry out dosage calculations accurately, I have tried to help them develop a sound base of safe practice.

A Nurse's Guide to Dosage Calculations: Giving Medications Safely was written to share my experience and expertise with nurses at all levels so that they will have a tool to help them do it "right."

Organization

This book is organized into units that follow the process by which you give medications. You must be able to do the basic math before you start. You then have to get the doctor's order and interpret it correctly. Once you know what medications you are supposed to give, you have to be able to calculate the correct dose. The next step is to prepare the medications for administration. Finally, some situations for which you need additional knowledge to carry out the procedures safely are explained.

Unit 1, Review the Math, provides a review of the basic math skills needed to carry out dosage calculations.

Unit 2, Interpret the Doctor's Order, discusses the theory base needed to understand medical orders. The abbreviations used in the clinical setting are defined and discussed. Chapter 4, Systems of Measurement, focuses primarily on the SI system, as this is the standard for health care in Canada. The apothecary and household systems are discussed very briefly, for those rare occasions when you may encounter them. Chapter 5, Components of a Doctor's Order, identifies all of the elements that have to be present in a doctor's order and the information you need to interpret each of those elements correctly. In Chapter 6, Interpreting Drug Labels, an explanation of all of the information on different types of drug labels is given. Chapter 7, Medication Systems, describes some of the common organizational systems found in health care settings.

Unit 3, Calculate the Dose, is the core of the book. Three methods of calculating dosages are presented for both oral and parenteral medications. Each of these methods is safe and appropriate, and none is better than the others. It is up to you to find the method that works best for you.

Unit 4, Administer the Medications, tells you how to prepare a variety of medications for administration. In addition to discussing oral and injectable medications, this unit covers all of the elements of IV administration. Chapter 12, Intravenous Therapy, and Chapter 13, Intravenous Medications, discuss the equipment and calculations needed for running IVs safely and for administering medications, as well as the use of subcutaneous infusion pumps.

Unit 5, Special Calculations, focuses on additional information you will need for specific occasions. These include paediatric calculations, the administration of insulin, heparin, blood and blood products, and parenteral nutrition.

Features

Several special features have been included in this book to help you practice safely. Each chapter begins with specific learning objectives, which are followed by a glossary of key terms used in that chapter. Keep It Safe and Make a Note boxes highlight some of the helpful tips and techniques I have developed over 20 years of teaching. Critical Thinking boxes present hypothetical situations for you to think about and perhaps discuss with your colleagues. I have not included answers to them, because there is no one right answer in these situations.

There are also a number of opportunities for you to practice the calculations presented in the book. After each calculation, the You Try It questions give you a chance to practice. The answers to these questions are at the end of the book. The steps in each calculation are written out, so that if you have a problem, you can see how it should have been done. At the end of most chapters, a Self Test covers all of the material in the chapter. The answers to the Self Tests are also at the end of the book. I hope these features are helpful to you in calculating and administering medications safely.

Vicki Niblett, RN, BScN

Find the Answer: A Quick Guide to the Calculations You Need

HOW DO I:

CONVERT VALUES IN THE METRIC SYSTEM?

milligrams (mg) to grams (g) — move the decimal point 3 places to the left
grams (g) to milligrams (mg) — move the decimal point 3 places to the right
micrograms (µg) to milligrams (mg) — move the decimal point 3 places to the left
milligrams (mg) to micrograms (µg) — move the decimal point 3 places to the right

See Chapter 4, page 47.

CALCULATE HOW MUCH DRUG TO GIVE?

Ratio and Proportion

See Chapter 8, page 95.

Formula

$$\frac{\text{Dose }\mathbf{D}\text{esired (mg)}}{\text{Dose on }\mathbf{H}\text{and (mg)}} \times \mathbf{S}\text{tock (tablets or ml)} = \mathbf{A}\text{mount (tablets or ml)}$$

$$\frac{\mathbf{D}}{\mathbf{H}} \times \mathbf{S} = \mathbf{A}$$

See Chapter 8, page 96.

CALCULATE IV FLOW RATES?

$$\frac{\text{Amount of fluid (ml)}}{\text{Time in hours}} = \text{Flow rate (ml/hr)}$$

See Chapter 12, page 145.

CALCULATE IV DRIP RATES FOR MACRO TUBING?

$$\frac{\text{Flow rate (ml/hour)}}{60 \text{ (minutes)}} \times \text{Drip factor (gtts/ml)} = \text{Drip rate (gtts/min)}$$

See Chapter 12, page 145.

or

$$\frac{\text{Amount of fluid } \times \text{ Drip factor}}{\text{Time in hours } \times \text{ 60 minutes}} = \text{Drip rate}$$

See Chapter 12, page 145.

CALCULATE IV DRIP RATES FOR MICRO TUBING?

Flow rate (ml/hr) = Drip rate (gtts/min)

See Chapter 12, page 148.

CALCULATE THE DRIP RATE FOR MINIBAG ADMINISTRATION OF IV MEDICATIONS?

$$\frac{\text{Amount of fluid (ml)} \times \text{Drip factor (gtts/ml)}}{\text{Time (minutes)}} = \text{Drip rate (gtts/min)}$$

See Chapter 13, page 157.

CALCULATE THE FLOW RATE FOR MINIBAGS USED WITH AN IV PUMP?

$$\frac{\text{Amount of solution (ml)}}{\text{Time (minutes)}} \times 60\ \text{(minutes)} = \text{Flow rate}$$

See Chapter 13, page 158.

CALCULATE THE DRIP RATES FOR SOLUSETS?

$$\frac{\text{Amount of solution (ml)}}{\text{Time (minutes)}} \times 60 = \text{Flow rate} = \text{Drip rate}$$

See Chapter 13, page 159.

CALCULATE THE FLOW RATE FOR DRUGS ORDERED AS mg/hr?

Set up a ratio and proportion where:
The **known ratio** is the concentration of drug (mg) : volume (ml)
The **unknown ratio** is hourly drug (mg) : hourly volume (ml) or flow rate
Use means = extremes or cross multiplication to solve for flow rate.

DRAW UP THE CORRECT AMOUNT OF TWO TYPES OF INSULIN IN THE SAME SYRINGE?

Calculate the total volume of insulin to be drawn up: Amount of cloudy + Amount of clear insulin.
Draw up an amount of air equal to the dose of **cloudy** insulin and inject it into the cloudy bottle.
Draw up an amount of air equal to the dose of **clear** insulin and inject it into the clear bottle.
Withdraw the appropriate dose of insulin from the **clear** bottle.
Insert the needle into the **cloudy** bottle and pull back on the plunger until the syringe is filled with the amount equal to the total calculated.

See Chapter 14, page 180.

CALCULATE THE DOSE OF DRUGS ORDERED IN DOSE/kg?

Dose of drug (µg/kg) × Body weight (kg) = Dose of drug (µg)

See Chapter 16, page 203.

CALCULATE BODY SURFACE AREA?

$$\text{BSA(m}^2) = \sqrt{\frac{\text{Weight (kg)} \times \text{Height (cm)}}{3\,600}}$$

If a body surface nomogram is available, draw a line from the patient's height (cm) on the left side of the scale to the patient's weight (kg) on the right side of the scale. The point at which this line intersects the middle scale is the body surface area (m^2).

See Chapter 16, page 206.

CALCULATE THE DOSE OF DRUGS ORDERED IN DOSE/m²?

Calculate the body surface area

Dose of drug mg/m^2 $\times$ BSA (m^2) $=$ mg of drug

See Chapter 16, page 208.

CALCULATE THE APPROPRIATE AMOUNT OF FLUID FOR A CHILD?

100 ml/kg/day for each kg up to 10 kg
plus
50 ml/kg/day for each additional kg up to 20 kg
plus
20 ml/kg/day for each additional kg

See Chapter 16, page 214.

Acknowledgments

I would like to thank my friends, colleagues, and family for their support and encouragement while I was writing this book. To the nursing faculty at Loyalist College of Applied Arts and Technology, thank you for listening to me and offering your suggestions. I would not have been able to carry out this project without the ongoing support of my Dean, Karen Brooks Cathcart. I would especially like to thank two special friends: Alison Kodatsky, my office mate of 15 years, for meticulous checking of the manuscript; and Marylin King, for vacuuming while I typed.

I would like to thank my son, Peter, for his encouragement and sense of humour, but most of all, I want to thank my husband, Mark. I truly could not have done this without his active support. Mark and I have been partners in this endeavour, as we have in everything else.

V. N.

Contents

means = extremes

Review the Math

150 mg: A ml: 50 mg: 2 ml

(g/ml)

75 mg: A ml: 100 mg: 1 ml

Basic Math Review

The student will:

- define the parts of a fraction
- identify the different types of fractions
- carry out selected operations with fractions
- correctly add, subtract, multiply, and divide fractions

- define decimals
- identify the rules for writing decimals
- identify the rules for rounding decimals
- correctly add, subtract, multiply, and divide decimals
- convert decimals to fractions and fractions to decimals

- define percent
- correctly convert decimals to percent and percent to decimals
- correctly convert fractions to percent and percent to fractions

Fraction: a number that represents a part of a whole number.

Numerator: the number of equal parts being represented; the "top" number.

Denominator: the total number of equal parts; the "bottom" number.

Proper fraction: fraction in which the numerator is less than the denominator.

Improper fraction: fraction in which the numerator is greater than the denominator.

Mixed number: a whole number plus a fraction.

Enlarging a fraction: multiplying both the numerator and the denominator by the same number.

Reducing a fraction: dividing both the numerator and the denominator by the same number.

Lowest common denominator: the lowest common number that can be divided evenly by the denominators of the fractions being compared.

Decimals: fractions in which the denominator is 10 or a multiple of 10.

Dividend: a number that is being divided.

Divisor: a number that is doing the dividing.

Quotient: the result of dividing a dividend by a divisor.

Percent: number of parts of a quantity per hundred.

Fractions

When something is divided into equal parts, we need a way of indicating how many of the parts we want to deal with. Fractions are the way that we do this. Fractions are written as two numbers, one number on top of the other with a line between them, such as $\frac{3}{4}$.

The top number, called the numerator, indicates the number of parts you want to consider. The bottom number, called the denominator, indicates the total number of parts.

If you have a pizza that is cut into four equal pieces, each piece is one part and would be indicated by a "1" in the numerator. The total number of pieces would be represented by a "4" in the denominator. Thus one piece of this pizza would be shown as $\frac{1}{4}$.

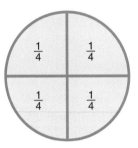

If you have two pieces of the pizza, you have $\frac{2}{4}$.

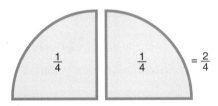

If you have three pieces, you have $\frac{3}{4}$.

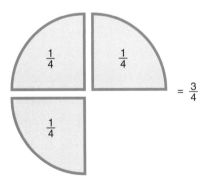

Fractions can be either proper fractions or improper fractions. In a proper fraction, the numerator is less than the denominator, such as $\frac{3}{4}$.

A proper fraction has fewer pieces than the whole.

An improper fraction is one in which the numerator is more than the denominator. In other words, you have more pieces than the whole, such as in $\frac{7}{4}$.

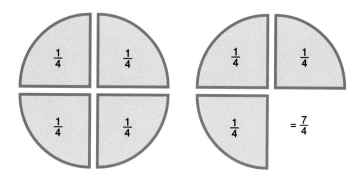

A mixed number consists of a whole number plus a fraction. To convert an improper fraction into a mixed number, divide the numerator by the denominator.

7 divided by 4 = 1 plus $\frac{3}{4}$

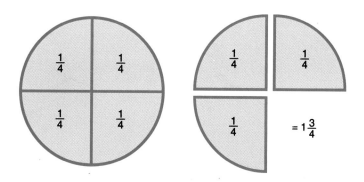

Similarly, mixed numbers can be converted into improper fractions by multiplying the whole number times the denominator and adding this result to the numerator. The denominator stays the same; only the numerator changes.

To change $1\frac{3}{4}$ to an improper fraction, multiply $4 \times 1 = 4$.

Add this to the numerator $4 + 3 = 7$.

The new numerator is 7. The fraction is $\frac{7}{4}$.

If both the numerator and the denominator of a fraction are multiplied or divided by the same number, the value of the fraction stays the same.

$$\frac{1\,(\times 2)}{4\,(\times 2)} = \frac{2}{8}$$

Multiplying both the numerator and the denominator of a fraction by the same number is called enlarging a fraction.

A fraction can be reduced if both the numerator and denominator can be divided evenly by the same number. For example, to reduce $\frac{6}{8}$ divide both the numerator and the denominator by 2.

$$\frac{6\,(\div 2)}{8\,(\div 2)} = \frac{3}{4}$$

Fractions are frequently easier to work with if they are reduced to the lowest denominator.

Comparing the Sizes of Fractions

When you are preparing medications, you sometimes need to determine which of two or more fractions is larger. If the denominators are the same, the fraction that has the larger numerator is the larger fraction.

$$\frac{3}{4} \text{ is larger than } \frac{1}{4}$$

If the numerators are the same, the fraction that has the smaller denominator is the larger fraction.

$$\frac{1}{4} \text{ is larger than } \frac{1}{8}$$

If both the numerator and the denominator are different, the fractions must be changed so that they have the same denominator. This is done by finding the lowest common denominator.

Finding the Lowest Common Denominator

To find the lowest common denominator of two fractions, you must find the lowest common number that can be divided evenly by both denominators. For example, with $\frac{5}{6}$ and $\frac{7}{8}$ the lowest common number that can be divided evenly by both 6 and 8 is 24. Both fractions must be changed so that they have a denominator of 24.

$$\text{To change } \frac{5}{6} \qquad 24 \div 6 = 4 \qquad \text{so } \frac{5\,(\times 4)}{6\,(\times 4)} = \frac{20}{24}$$

$$\text{To change } \frac{7}{8} \qquad 24 \div 8 = 3 \qquad \text{so } \frac{7\,(\times 3)}{8\,(\times 3)} = \frac{21}{24}$$

Now that both fractions have the same denominator, they can be compared.

$$\frac{21}{24} \text{ is larger than } \frac{20}{24}, \text{ so } \frac{7}{8} \text{ is larger than } \frac{5}{6}$$

If the denominator of one fraction can be divided evenly by the denominator of the other fraction, it is only necessary to change the smaller one. For example, in $\frac{7}{10}$ and $\frac{3}{5}$, 10 can be evenly divided by 5, so it is only necessary to change $\frac{3}{5}$.

$$10 \div 5 = 2 \text{ so } \frac{3\,(\times 2)}{5\,(\times 2)} = \frac{6}{10}$$

Now the two fractions can be compared:

$$\frac{7}{10} \text{ is larger than } \frac{6}{10}, \text{ so } \frac{7}{10} \text{ is larger than } \frac{3}{5}$$

MAKE A NOTE ✔

There is no rule or procedure for finding the number that can be evenly divided by the denominators. The process is one of trial and error. There are, however, some guidelines:

Even numbers can be divided by 2 and sometimes by multiples of 2.

Numbers ending in 5 or 0 can be divided by 5.

The numbers 2, 3, 5, 7, and 11 are prime numbers and cannot be divided, but other odd numbers can sometimes be divided by them.

YOU TRY IT

(The answers to these questions are found at the end of the book.)

MANIPULATING FRACTIONS

1. Change the following improper fractions to mixed numbers.

   1. $\dfrac{7}{3}$ 2. $\dfrac{6}{4}$ 3. $\dfrac{23}{9}$ 4. $\dfrac{30}{5}$ 5. $\dfrac{17}{6}$

2. Change the following mixed numbers to improper fractions.

   6. $2\dfrac{7}{8}$ 7. $1\dfrac{1}{4}$ 8. $6\dfrac{9}{16}$ 9. $10\dfrac{23}{25}$ 10. $3\dfrac{3}{5}$

3. Find the lowest common denominator for the following pairs of fractions and identify which of the fractions is larger.

   11. $\dfrac{4}{7}$ and $\dfrac{6}{11}$ 12. $\dfrac{4}{5}$ and $\dfrac{9}{10}$ 13. $\dfrac{7}{9}$ and $\dfrac{3}{4}$

   14. $\dfrac{5}{8}$ and $\dfrac{7}{10}$ 15. $\dfrac{2}{3}$ and $\dfrac{4}{6}$

Adding and Subtracting Fractions

In order to add or subtract fractions, the denominators must be the same. If both are the same, add or subtract the numerators and place the result over the denominator. It is usually easier to work with the numbers if you then reduce the fraction to its lowest common denominator.

$$\text{e.g., } \frac{3}{10} + \frac{5}{10} = \frac{8}{10}$$

By dividing both the numerator and the denominator by 2, $\frac{8}{10}$ can be reduced:

$$\frac{8\ (\div 2)}{10\ (\div 2)} = \frac{4}{5}$$

If the denominators are different, you must first find the lowest common denominator for all of the fractions you have to add. Once they all have a common denominator, you proceed as above.

$$\text{e.g., } \frac{2}{3} + \frac{4}{5} + \frac{5}{6} =$$

The lowest common denominator for 3, 5, and 6 is 30. Each fraction must be changed so it has a denominator of 30.

To change $\frac{2}{3}$ to 30ths: $30 \div 3 = 10$ so $\frac{2\ (\times 10)}{3\ (\times 10)} = \frac{20}{30}$

To change $\frac{4}{5}$ to 30ths: $30 \div 5 = 6$ so $\frac{4\ (\times 6)}{5\ (\times 6)} = \frac{24}{30}$

To change $\frac{5}{6}$ to 30ths: $30 \div 6 = 5$ so $\frac{5\ (\times 5)}{6\ (\times 5)} = \frac{25}{30}$

You can then add $\frac{20}{30} + \frac{24}{30} + \frac{25}{30} = \frac{69}{30}$

Reduce $\frac{69}{30}$ to $2\frac{9}{30}$ or $2\frac{3}{10}$

The best way to add mixed numbers is to change them to improper fractions; find the lowest common denominator; add the fractions; and then change the result back into a mixed number.

YOU TRY IT

(The answers to these questions are found at the end of the book.)

ADDING AND SUBTRACTING FRACTIONS

Reduce the answer to the lowest common denominator.

1. $\frac{3}{4} - \frac{2}{3}$

2. $\frac{4}{5} + \frac{6}{8} + \frac{7}{10}$

3. $3\frac{3}{4} + \frac{3}{5} + \frac{3}{6}$

4. $7\frac{1}{2} - 5\frac{3}{5}$

5. $6\frac{4}{6} + 3\frac{5}{9} + 7\frac{7}{12}$

Multiplying Fractions

To multiply fractions, multiply the numerators to get the new numerator. Multiply the denominators to get the new denominator. If possible, reduce the fraction to the lowest common denominator.

$$\text{e.g.,} \ \frac{3}{4} \times \frac{5}{6} = \frac{15}{24}$$

Don't worry about multiplying mixed numbers, just convert the mixed number to an improper fraction and then proceed as above.

YOU TRY IT

(The answers to these questions are found at the end of the book.)

MULTIPLYING FRACTIONS

Reduce the answer to the lowest denominator.

1. $\dfrac{4}{9} \times \dfrac{7}{12}$ 2. $\dfrac{6}{10} \times \dfrac{11}{12}$ 3. $\dfrac{55}{60} \times \dfrac{92}{100}$

4. $\dfrac{12}{36} \times \dfrac{15}{30}$ 5. $\dfrac{13}{15} \times \dfrac{17}{19}$

Dividing Fractions

To divide fractions, invert (turn upside down) the fraction after the division sign and change the division sign to a multiplication sign.

$$\frac{7}{8} \div \frac{2}{3} = \frac{7}{8} \times \frac{3}{2} = \frac{21}{16} = 1\frac{5}{16}$$

YOU TRY IT

(The answers to these questions are found at the end of the book.)

DIVIDING FRACTIONS

Reduce the answer to the lowest common denominator.

1. $\dfrac{4}{9} \div \dfrac{7}{12}$ 2. $\dfrac{6}{10} \div \dfrac{11}{12}$ 3. $\dfrac{55}{60} \div \dfrac{92}{100}$

4. $\dfrac{12}{36} \div \dfrac{15}{30}$ 5. $\dfrac{13}{15} \div \dfrac{17}{19}$

Decimal System

The decimal system consists of whole numbers and fractions in which the denominator is 10 or a multiple of 10. Rather than writing the fraction as a numerator and denominator, a decimal point is used to distinguish between whole numbers and fractions. Whole numbers appear to the left of the decimal point, while decimal fractions appear to the right. The value of an individual numeral depends on its position within a number. Each place to the left of the decimal point is 10 times greater than the numeral to its right. Each place to the right of the decimal point is 1/10 the value of the numeral to its left.

$$1\,000 \quad 100 \quad 10 \quad 1 \qquad \frac{1}{10} \quad \frac{1}{100} \quad \frac{1}{1\,000} \quad \frac{1}{10\,000}$$

thousands   hundreds   tens   ones   .   tenths   hundredths   thousandths   ten-thousandths

MAKE A NOTE

Numerals to the left of a decimal point have a value of 1 or more.

Numerals to the right of a decimal point have a value of less than 1.

There are some conventions, or rules, that make dealing with decimals easier:

- When there is no whole number to the left of a decimal point, a zero should be placed to the left of the decimal point. This makes it easy to identify a number as a decimal fraction.
- There should not be a zero at the end of a decimal fraction. While the zero does not change the value of the number, it can increase confusion. Zeros may be added temporarily to make addition or subtraction easier, but they should be removed when stating the final answer.

MAKE A NOTE

When you are comparing decimal numbers, it is important to be able to figure out which one is larger and which is smaller:

If the decimal numbers contain different whole numbers, the one with the higher whole number is the larger number.

6.4 is larger than 3.7

If the whole numbers are the same, or there are no whole numbers, the decimal with the higher number in the tenths place is the larger number.

0.46 is larger than 0.28

If the numbers in the tenths places are the same or 0, the decimal with the higher number in the hundredths place is the larger, and so on.

0.05 is larger than 0.025

Rounding Off Decimals

Some calculations will produce results in which the number of places to the right of the decimal point is very large, or in some cases, infinite. These can be very unwieldy to work with, so decimals are usually rounded off to an appropriate number of places. The number of places is dependent on the use of the decimals. When preparing medications, decimals are usually rounded off to either tenths (0.1) or hundredths (0.01).

To round off a decimal, decide how many decimal places you want. Look at the numeral immediately to the right of the last decimal place you want to keep. If it is 5 or larger, add 1 to the last number you are keeping and erase the rest. If the numeral immediately to the right is less than 5, erase the numbers without adding anything to the remainder.

e.g., round off 12.37634 to two decimal places
The last numeral you want to keep is 7
The numeral to the right of the 7 is 6
This is larger than 5, so you will add 1 to 7
The number is rounded off to 12.38

YOU TRY IT

(The answers to these questions are found at the end of the book.)

ROUNDING OFF DECIMALS

1. Round off 17.638 to 2 decimal places.

2. Round off 4.0028 to 2 decimal places.

3. Round off 0.4555 to 3 decimal places.

4. Round off 3.3333333333 to 2 decimal places.

5. Round off 0.25 to 1 decimal place.

Adding and Subtracting Decimal Fractions

Adding and subtracting decimal fractions is similar to adding and subtracting whole numbers. The important difference is that the decimal points must be lined up so that tenths are being added to tenths and hundredths are being added to hundredths, etc.

e.g.,   12.76 + 3.04 + 0.455

Set this up in columns to make it easier, but be sure that the decimal points are lined up.

```
  12.76
   3.04
+  0.455
 16.255
```

When you are subtracting decimal fractions, it is helpful to temporarily add zeros to the right side of some numbers for ease of calculation.

e.g.,   15.74 − 12.836

Set up the columns, and add a zero to 15.74 to make it easier.

```
  15.740
 −12.836
   2.904
```

YOU TRY IT

(The answers to these questions are found at the end of the book.)

ADDING AND SUBTRACTING DECIMALS

1. 51.06 + 19.44 + 21.73

2. 14.75 + 12.25

3. 22.33 + 44.33 + 66.33

4. 12.575 + 75.05 + 9.4

5. 30.03 + 19.02 + 12.375

6. 54.09 − 22.36

7. 33.33 − 30.003

8. 65.011 − 12.2

9. 48.67 − 39.4

10. 68.77 − 54.098

Multiplying Decimals

It is not necessary to line up the decimal points when multiplying. Carry out the multiplication as if there were no decimal points present. When you get the answer, count the number of decimal places in both numbers. Put the total number of decimal places into the resulting number.

e.g., $24.3 \times 7.8 = 189.54$

There is one decimal place in each of the numbers being multiplied, so there are two decimal places in the answer.

YOU TRY IT

(The answers to these questions are found at the end of the book.)

MULTIPLYING DECIMALS

Round off the answer to two decimal places.

1. 16.44×14.3 2. 5.75×15.5 3. 42.77×33.33

4. 6.66×12.5 5. 20.02×4.11

Dividing Decimals

In order to understand division of decimals, it is helpful to know the names of the parts of a division problem.

Dividend is the number that is being divided.
Divisor is the number that is doing the dividing.
Quotient is the answer.

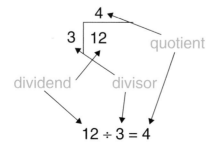

To divide decimals, the decimal point in the divisor is moved to the right until it is a whole number. The decimal point in the dividend is then moved the same number of places to the right. The decimal point in the quotient is placed directly above the decimal point in the dividend.

e.g., $16.45 \div 3.75 =$

$$16.456 \div 3.75$$

$$16.456 \div 3.75$$

$$1\ 645.6 \div 375 = 4.388$$

Dividing decimals can result in quotients that extend to a very large number of decimal places. You should decide how many decimal places you want and follow the rules about rounding off decimals for your answer.

YOU TRY IT

(The answers to these questions are found at the end of the book.)

DIVIDING DECIMALS

Round off the answer to two decimal places.

1. $56.45 \div 2.4$ 2. $133.3 \div 15.75$ 3. $675 \div 0.125$

4. $336.6 \div 13.2$ 5. $455.8 \div 22.25$

Multiplying and Dividing Decimals by 10

Decimals are multiples and fractions of 10. This makes it very easy to multiply and divide by 10.

To multiply a decimal by 10, move the decimal point one place to the right.

e.g., $0.03 \times 10 = 0.3$

To multiply a decimal by a multiple of 10 (100, 1 000, 10 000, etc.), move the decimal point to the right the same number of places as there are zeros in the number you are multiplying by.

e.g., $2.3437 \times 1\ 000 = 2\ 343.7$

To divide a decimal by 10, move the decimal point one place to the left.

e.g., $0.03 : 10 = 0.003$

To divide a decimal by a multiple of 10 (100, 1 000, 10 000, etc.), move the decimal point to the left the same number of places as there are zeros in the number you are dividing by.

e.g., $2.3437 : 1\ 000 = 0.0023437$

MAKE A NOTE ✓

Moving a decimal point to the right makes a number larger.

Moving a decimal point to the left makes a number smaller.

Converting Decimals to Fractions

To convert a decimal to a fraction, recall that the decimal point is taking the place of the denominator: 1.25 can be stated as 1 and 25 one-hundredths. Count the number of places to the right of the decimal point. This will be the number of zeros in the denominator of the fraction.

e.g., $4.75 = 4\dfrac{75}{100}$

YOU TRY IT

(The answers to these questions are found at the end of the book.)

CONVERTING DECIMALS TO FRACTIONS

Convert the following decimals to fractions. Reduce the fractions to the lowest common denominator.

1. 3.33   2. 6.66   3. 0.458   4. 0.083   5. 0.625

Converting Fractions to Decimals

To convert a fraction to a decimal, divide the numerator by the denominator. Place the decimal point immediately to the right of the numerator. Add zeros after the decimal point as necessary to make the problem easier to work. You should decide how many decimal places you want for the answer and round it off appropriately.

e.g., $\dfrac{5}{8} =$

$$5.000 \div 8 = 0.625$$

If the fraction is a mixed number, convert it to an improper fraction before carrying out the division.

YOU TRY IT

(The answers to these questions are found at the end of the book.)

CONVERTING FRACTIONS TO DECIMALS

Convert the following fractions to decimals. State the answer to two decimal places.

1. $\dfrac{2}{3}$ 2. $\dfrac{6}{8}$ 3. $\dfrac{25}{45}$ 4. $\dfrac{93}{125}$ 5. $\dfrac{468}{500}$

Percents

Percent is another method of expressing fractions. It is represented by the % sign and means hundredths. As a fraction, the denominator is 100. As a decimal, it is two decimal places.

e.g., $5\% = \dfrac{5}{100} = 0.05$

Converting Between Decimals and Percent

To change a decimal to percent, move the decimal point two places to the right and add the percent sign.

e.g., $0.025 = 2.5\%$

To change a percent to a decimal, remove the percent sign and move the decimal point two places to the left.

e.g., $15\% = 0.15$

YOU TRY IT

(The answers to these questions are found at the end of the book.)

CONVERTING BETWEEN DECIMALS AND PERCENT

Convert the following decimals to percent:

1. 0.13   2. 4.375   3. 33.3   4. 0.09   5. 0.88

Convert the following percents to decimals:

6. 72%   7. 0.3%   8. 92.4%   9. 0.09%   10. 66.6%

Converting Between Fractions and Percent

To change a fraction to a percent, change the fraction to a decimal, then change the decimal to a percent.

e.g., Convert $\dfrac{2}{3}$ to a percent.

Change $\dfrac{2}{3}$ to a decimal

Divide 2 by 3:

$2 \div 3 = 0.67$

Change 0.67 to a percent by moving the decimal point two places to the right and adding the percent sign:

$0.67 = 67\%$

To change a percent to a fraction, change the percent to a decimal, then change the decimal to a fraction.

e.g., Convert 25% to a fraction

Change 25% to a decimal by removing the percent sign and moving the decimal point two places to the left:

$25\% = 0.25$

Change 0.25 to a fraction:

$0.25 = \dfrac{25}{100}$

Reduce the fraction:

$\dfrac{25}{100} = \dfrac{1}{4}$

YOU TRY IT

(The answers to these questions are found at the end of the book.)

CONVERTING BETWEEN FRACTIONS AND PERCENT

Convert the following fractions to percent:

1. $\dfrac{3}{4}$ 2. $\dfrac{28}{36}$ 3. $\dfrac{55}{64}$ 4. $\dfrac{18}{20}$ 5. $\dfrac{45}{50}$

Convert the following percents to fractions and reduce the fraction to the lowest common denominator:

1. 40%   2. 185%   3. 75%   4. 66%   5. 31%

Self Test

The answers to these questions are found at the end of the book.

Change the following improper fractions to mixed numbers. Reduce the answer to the lowest common denominator.

1. $\dfrac{22}{17}$　　　2. $\dfrac{15}{12}$　　　3. $\dfrac{9}{8}$　　　4. $\dfrac{60}{55}$　　　5. $\dfrac{66}{30}$

Change the following mixed numbers to improper fractions. Reduce the answer to the lowest common denominator.

6. $1\dfrac{6}{9}$　　　7. $4\dfrac{22}{25}$　　　8. $5\dfrac{24}{30}$　　　9. $17\dfrac{14}{15}$　　　10. $44\dfrac{3}{4}$

For each of the following pairs of fractions, identify which of the two fractions is larger.

11. $\dfrac{3}{4}$ and $\dfrac{5}{8}$　　　12. $\dfrac{22}{25}$ and $\dfrac{15}{20}$　　　13. $\dfrac{6}{9}$ and $\dfrac{9}{12}$　　　14. $\dfrac{12}{15}$ and $\dfrac{10}{13}$　　　15. $\dfrac{22}{25}$ and $\dfrac{27}{30}$

Add the following fractions. Reduce the answer to the lowest common denominator.

16. $3\dfrac{1}{4} + \dfrac{2}{5}$ 17. $\dfrac{6}{9} + \dfrac{9}{12}$ 18. $\dfrac{3}{8} + 15\dfrac{11}{12}$ 19. $\dfrac{22}{30} + \dfrac{5}{6}$ 20. $\dfrac{5}{8} + \dfrac{7}{9}$

Subtract the following fractions. Reduce the answer to the lowest common denominator.

21. $2\dfrac{3}{8} - 1\dfrac{4}{7} =$ 22. $5\dfrac{6}{7} - 2\dfrac{5}{9} =$ 23. $\dfrac{4}{5} - \dfrac{3}{8} =$

24. $6\dfrac{11}{12} - 2\dfrac{15}{18} =$ 25. $4\dfrac{6}{9} - 3\dfrac{4}{6} =$

Multiply the following fractions. Reduce the answer to the lowest common denominator.

26. $\dfrac{8}{9} \times \dfrac{12}{16} =$ 27. $\dfrac{15}{18} \times \dfrac{12}{13} =$ 28. $4\dfrac{6}{10} \times \dfrac{17}{19} =$

29. $\dfrac{18}{20} \times \dfrac{1}{2} =$ 30. $5\dfrac{2}{3} \times \dfrac{15}{18} =$

Divide the following fractions. Reduce the answer to the lowest common denominator.

31. $\dfrac{8}{9} \div \dfrac{12}{16} =$ 32. $\dfrac{15}{18} \div \dfrac{12}{13} =$ 33. $4\dfrac{6}{10} \div \dfrac{17}{19} =$

34. $\dfrac{18}{20} \div \dfrac{1}{2} =$ 35. $5\dfrac{2}{3} \div \dfrac{15}{18} =$

Convert the following decimals to fractions. Reduce the answer to the lowest common denominator.

36. 1.125   37. 5.67   38. 15.75   39. 0.225   40. 0.043

Convert the following fractions to decimals. State the answer to two decimal places.

41. $\dfrac{1}{2}$ 42. $\dfrac{3}{4}$ 43. $\dfrac{1}{10}$ 44. $\dfrac{13}{15}$ 45. $\dfrac{39}{40}$

Convert the following decimals to percent. State the answer to one decimal place.

46. 0.25   47. 1.75   48. 0.03   49. 2.04   50. 0.009

Convert the following percents to decimals.

51. 3.33%   52. 0.3%   53. 0.9%   54. 50%   55. 5.25%

Convert the following fractions to percents. State the answer to one decimal place.

56. $\dfrac{1}{3}$ 57. $\dfrac{1}{8}$ 58. $\dfrac{1}{6}$ 59. $\dfrac{2}{3}$ 60. $\dfrac{3}{5}$

Convert the following percents to fractions. Reduce the fraction to its lowest common denominator.

61. 20%   62. 48%   63. 54%   64. 71%   65. 24%

Calculations Used in Determining Drug Doses

The student will:

- define ratio
- identify the ratio when given two quantities or numbers

- define proportion
- use proportion to solve for an unknown quantity by the following methods:
  - **Means = Extremes**
  - **cross multiplication**

- define formula
- substitute the appropriate numbers and units in a given formula

Ratio: an expression of the relationship between two numbers or two quantities.

Proportion: the relationship between two equal ratios.

Formula: a statement of the procedure for calculating a desired value or result.

One of the key elements in giving medications safely is solving a problem for an unknown quantity. Ratio and Proportion is one way of doing this. We will look at two different ways of solving for an unknown using ratio and proportion in this chapter.

Ratios

A ratio is an expression of the relationship between two numbers or two quantities. A slash (/) or a colon (:) divides the two numbers and is read as "is to" or "per." If a family has one boy and two girls, the ratio of boys to girls is 1/2, or 1:2.

✔ MAKE A NOTE

When you are using ratios, make sure you are comparing the correct quantities.

If you have a box of 25 candies and 10 of them are chocolate and 15 are vanilla, the ratio of chocolate candies to vanilla candies is 10/15, or 10:15; the ratio of chocolate candies to all of the candies is 10/25, or 10:25.

YOU TRY IT

(The answers to these questions are found at the end of the book.)

RATIOS

1. You have 15 carrots and 20 potatoes. What is the ratio of carrots to potatoes?

2. Your term test has 40 questions. You answered 35 correctly. What is the ratio of questions answered correctly to the total number of questions? What is the ratio of incorrect answers to correct answers?

3. Your cat has just had seven kittens. Three are black, two are white, one is grey, and one is orange. What is the ratio of black kittens to the total number of kittens? What is the ratio of white kittens to black kittens? What is the ratio of grey kittens to black kittens?

4. You are making fruit salad. The recipe calls for 2 cups of blueberries and 3 cups of strawberries. What is the ratio of blueberries to strawberries?

5. You are buying snacks for a party. You buy 12 bags of potato chips and 6 bags of taco chips. What is the ratio of taco chips to potato chips? What is the ratio of potato chips to the total number of bags of snacks?

Proportion

Proportion is the relationship between two equal ratios. It can be written three different ways:

separated by an equal sign $3 : 5 = 6 : 10$

as a fraction $\dfrac{3}{5} = \dfrac{6}{10}$

separated by a double colon $3 : 5 :: 6 : 10$

They all mean that the relationship between 3 and 5 is the same as the relationship between 6 and 10.

Ratio and Proportion: Means = Extremes

When the ratio is written $3:5 = 6:10$, the product of multiplying the inner two numbers, the means, will equal the product of multiplying the outer two numbers, the extremes.

$$\downarrow\text{-means-}\downarrow$$

$$3:5 \quad = \quad 6:10$$

$$\uparrow\text{----extremes-----}\uparrow$$

Multiply the means $5 \times 6 = 30$
Multiply the extremes $3 \times 10 = 30$
Means = Extremes

This characteristic of ratio and proportion can be used to solve for an unknown when we have one known ratio and one unknown ratio.

EXAMPLE 2.1

You have a box of candy in which 12 of every 25 candies are chocolate. The box has 100 candies in it, so how many chocolate candies are in the box?

Write out the known ratio   12 chocolates : 25 candies
Write out the unknown ratio X chocolates : 100 candies
The relationship between the known ratio and the unknown ratio is the same, so

$$12 \text{ chocolates} : 25 \text{ candies} = X \text{ chocolates} : 100 \text{ candies}$$

When we look at the above proportion, the parts of the proportion closest to the equal sign are called the *means*. The parts at either end are called the *extremes*. The product of the means is equal to the product of the extremes.

$$\downarrow\text{----means----}\downarrow$$

$$12 \text{ chocolates} : 25 \text{ candies} = X \text{ chocolates} : 100 \text{ candies}$$

$$\uparrow\text{--------------------extremes--------------------}\uparrow$$

Means = $25 \times X = 25X$
Extremes = $12 \times 100 = 1200$

Means = Extremes
$25X = 1\,200$

$X = 1\,200 \div 25 = 48$

There are 48 chocolate candies in each box of 100 candies.

YOU TRY IT

(The answers to these questions are found at the end of the book.)

RATIO AND PROPORTION: MEANS = EXTREMES

1. The staffing ratio on your hospital unit is 1 nurse for each 6 patients. If there are 36 patients on the floor, how many nurses will there be?

2. You are making a stew. The recipe calls for 5 carrots for each potato that you put in. You decide to put in 15 carrots. How many potatoes will you put in?

3. The pet store usually has 3 dogs for every 2 cats in the store. If there are 21 dogs, how many cats are there?

4. The magazine has 5 pages of advertising for every 3 pages of news articles. If the magazine has 35 pages of advertising, how many pages of news articles does it have?

5. The radio station plays 7 commercials for every 2 songs that it plays. If it plays 6 songs in an hour, how many commercials will it play?

Ratio and Proportion: Cross Multiplication of Fractions

When the proportion is written as fractions $\dfrac{3}{5} = \dfrac{6}{10}$, the product of multiplying the numerator of one fraction by the denominator of the other fraction is equal to the product of multiplying the other numerator by the other denominator. This is called *cross multiplication.*

$$\dfrac{3}{5} \nwarrow \nearrow \dfrac{6}{10}$$

$$3 \times 10 = 30$$

$$5 \times 6 = 30$$

EXAMPLE 2.2

You're filling loot bags for a little boy's birthday party. You decide to put 10 little gifts in each bag. You will put in 3 erasers, 2 pencils, 2 notebooks, and 3 miniature cars in each bag. You will need 7 loot bags. How many erasers will you have to buy? The known ratio is 3 erasers in 1 loot bag.

$$\dfrac{3}{1}$$

The unknown ratio is X erasers in 7 loot bags:

$$\dfrac{X}{7}$$

The unknown ratio equals the known ratio:

$$\dfrac{X}{7} = \dfrac{3}{1}$$

Cross multiply the fractions:

$$\dfrac{X}{7} \nwarrow \nearrow \dfrac{3}{1}$$

$$X = 21$$

You will buy 21 erasers.

YOU TRY IT

(The answers to these questions are found at the end of the book.)

You are making a fruit punch for a minor hockey league banquet. The original recipe calls for 1 000 ml of cranberry cocktail, 750 ml of white grape juice, 500 ml of pineapple juice, 125 ml of lemon juice, and 750 ml of soda water. This will make 3 125 ml of punch. You estimate that you will need 25 000 ml (25 litres) for the banquet.

1. How many ml of cranberry cocktail will you need?

2. How many ml of white grape juice will you need?

3. How many ml of pineapple juice will you need?

4. How many ml of lemon juice will you need?

5. There are 500 ml of lemon juice in each bottle. How many bottles of lemon juice will you need?

Formula

A formula is a statement of the procedure for calculating a desired value or result.

EXAMPLE 2.3

To calculate the area of a rectangle, multiply the length times the width.

Length × Width = Area

Calculate the area of the rectangle in Figure 2.1:

Length is 4 cm
Width is 2 cm
Area is unknown

Length × Width = 4 cm × 2 cm = 8 square cm

The area of the rectangle is 8 square cm.

When a formula is written out in words, it can become somewhat unwieldy, so a letter or symbol is usually used to represent each word. The most common way to represent the words is to use the first letter of each word:

Length × Width = Area or L × W = A

When you are using a formula, it is important that you use the correct units for the quantities you are calculating. Similar types of quantities must use the same units. In the above example, both length and width are distances, so both must be in centimetres.

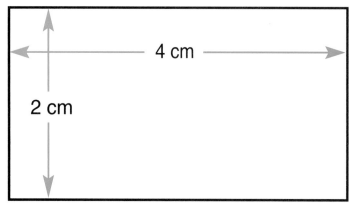

FIGURE 2-1

The result, or area, is a combination of the two units, in this case, square centimetres. (centimetre × centimetre is usually written as square centimetres.) If length were stated as 0.04 metres and the width as 2 cm, it would be necessary to convert them both to metres or both to centimetres.

Once you know a formula, you can solve for any unknown component. For example, if you know that a room is 12 square metres and that the width of the room is 3 metres, you can use the formula to calculate the length:

L × W = A

L × 3 metres = 12 square metres

$$\mathbf{L} = \frac{12\ \text{square metres}}{3\ \text{metres}}$$

L = 4 metres

MAKE A NOTE ✔

When you are putting the numbers into a formula, it is important that you also put in the units. Carry out your calculations and add the appropriate units to the answer as well. Those units that were in the numerator stay above the line and those in the denominator stay below the line.

For example, in order to calculate velocity (speed), divide the distance travelled by the time spent in travelling:

$$\mathbf{V}\text{elocity} = \frac{\mathbf{D}\text{istance}}{\mathbf{T}\text{ime}} \quad \text{or} \quad \mathbf{V} = \frac{\mathbf{D}}{\mathbf{T}}$$

If it took 3 hours to drive 330 km, what was the velocity?

$$\mathbf{V} = \frac{330\ \text{km}}{3\ \text{hours}}$$

V = 110 km/hour

Self Test

The answers to these questions are found at the end of the book.

You are making a snack mix to take to the hockey banquet. The recipe calls for the following:

125 ml of mixed nuts
200 ml of peanuts
250 ml of garlic-flavoured bite-size bagel chips
750 ml of waffle-shaped corn cereal
500 ml of waffle-shaped wheat cereal
1 000 ml of waffle-shaped rice cereal
90 ml of butter, melted
30 ml of Worcestershire sauce
10 ml of garlic powder
7.5 ml of seasoned salt
2.5 m. of onion powder

Heat the oven to 250°F.
Mix all of the ingredients in a large roast pan.
Bake 1 hour, stirring every 15 minutes.
Spread on paper towels to cool.
Makes 3 000 ml (3 litres) of snack mix.

You decide that you will need 12 000 ml (12 litres) of snack mix for the banquet.

Calculate how much of each of the following ingredients you will need for 12 000 ml of snack mix. Show your calculations using ratio and proportion: means = extremes and ratio and proportion: cross multiplication of fractions.

1. mixed nuts

2. peanuts

3. bagel chips

4. corn cereal

5. wheat cereal

6. rice cereal

7. butter

8. Worcestershire sauce

9. garlic powder

10. seasoned salt

11. onion powder

Interpret the Doctor's Order

Abbreviations

The student will:

- correctly identify abbreviations used by physicians and other health professionals writing medication orders:
  - drug preparations
  - routes
  - times
  - other

Medication orders are usually written using a number of abbreviations. It is expected that the nurse will know what these abbreviations mean and will be able to interpret them correctly. The following is a list of some of the more common ones. Many institutions have their own policy about abbreviations. Should there be an agency policy, you would of course use those.

✔ **MAKE A NOTE**

Medical abbreviations are written without periods. For example intramuscular *is abbreviated as IM, not I.M. The periods are omitted because they may be mistaken for a "1" if written in a hurry.*

Drug Preparations

amp	ampoule or ampule
cap	capsule or caplet
el or elix	elixir
ext	extract
fld	fluid
gtt	drop
liq	liquid
sol	solution
sp	spirit
sup or supp	suppository
susp	suspension
syr	syrup
tab	tablet
tr or tinct	tincture
ung or oint	ointment

Extended Action Drug Preparations

There are a number of drugs that are prepared so that they act over an extended period of time. Unfortunately there is no standard designation for these drugs. The following are some of the abbreviations used to indicate extended action, usually added to the end of the drug name, e.g., *Cardizem CD.*

Contin	Continuous release	Usually used with narcotic analgesics, e.g., MS Contin, morphine sulphate, continuous release
CD	Continuous dose or continuous delivery	
CR	Continuous release	
LA	Long acting	
SA	Sustained action	
SR	Sustained release or slow release	

KEEP IT SAFE Extended action medications are usually administered once or twice in 24 hours. The amount of medication in one dose is significantly higher than in the usual form. You should question the order calling for more frequent doses, and be comfortable with the reason before administering them.

Extended action medications are not broken or crushed unless they are capsules containing granules that can be mixed with food. Always consult the manufacturer's insert, the CPS, or a nursing drug guide before breaking open an extended action capsule.

Routes of Administration

The routes of administration are usually uppercase, though it is not unusual for them to be written in lowercase. Many of the older routes of administration are an abbreviation of the Latin terminology formerly used by physicians. The original Latin is included here for those who find it interesting.

AD	right ear	auris dextra
AS	left ear	auris sinistra
AU	both ears	aures uterque
ET	endotrachial tube	
IM	intramuscular	
IV	intravenous	
MDI	metered dose inhaler	
NGT or NG	nasogastric tube	
OD	right eye	oculus dexter
OS	left eye	oculus sinister
OU	both eyes	oculus uterque
Per	by	
PO	by mouth	per os
PR	in the rectum	per rectum
PV	in the vagina	per vagina
SC or Sub Q or SQ	subcutaneous	
SL	sublingual (under the tongue)	
ID	intradermal	
Neb	nebulizer	

Times of Administration

Times of administration are usually written in lowercase, but sometimes appear in uppercase. The Latin roots of these times are also included here.

ac	before meals	ante cibum
ad lib	as desired, freely	ad libitum
am	morning	ante meridium
bid	two times per day	bis en die
hs	bed time or evening	hora somni
od	each day	
pc	after meals	post cibum
prn	if necessary	pro re nata
q	each or every (q is usually combined with the frequency of administration)	quaque

q2h, q3h, etc.	every 2 hours, every 3 hours, etc.	quaque 2 hora, quaque 3 hora
qd	each day	
qam	every morning	quaque ante meridian
qhs	every evening	quaque hora somni
qid	four times per day	quater in die (note that in this case, q does not mean each)
stat	immediately	statim
tid	three times per day	ter in die
X	for, as in X 3 doses—for 3 doses	

✔ MAKE A NOTE

OD (right eye) and od (each day) are easily confused. While uppercase theoretically means the route and lowercase means the time, you cannot depend on this. The best way of telling them apart is by the context in which they are used.

The route is usually associated with medications that are in drop or ointment form. If the order already includes a time, OD or od probably means the route. If the order already includes a route, OD or od probably means the time. If the order is unclear, check with the person who wrote the order.

Miscellaneous

These are some miscellaneous abbreviations that are helpful to know when preparing to administer medications.

<	less than	
>	greater than	
$\bar{c}$	with	
d/c or dc	discontinue (depending on the context, it may mean discharge)	
KVO or TKVO	keep vein open; or to keep vein open	
n/a	not applicable	
nka	no known allergies	
NPO	nothing by mouth	nil per os
qs	quantity sufficient	
$\bar{s}$	without	
$\overline{ss}$	one half	
TPN	total parenteral nutrition	
$\bar{i}, \bar{ii}$	one, two	lowercase roman numerals with a line over them indicate the number of tablets or drops of a medication to be given

Self Test

Answers to these questions are found at the end of the book.

Write out each of the following in full:

1. Tylenol (acetaminophen) elix 80 mg per NG q4h prn.

2. Cardizem CD (diltiazem) 160 mg po qam.

3. Ativan 0.5 mg sl qhs.

4. Voltaren Opthalmic 1% sol (diclofenac) gtts i OS qid X 1 week then bid X 1 week.

5. Alti-Beclomethasone (beclomethasone) MDI 2 puffs q8h.

6. Dilaudid (hydromorphone) 4 mg IM q3h prn

Write out each of the following using the abbreviations in Chapter 3.

7. Canesten (nystatin) suppository 1 gram into the vagina at bedtime.

8. Nu-Ranit (ranitidine) 150 milligrams by mouth twice daily.

9. Ceruminex (triethanolamine polypeptide oleate-condensate) 1 millilitre in each ear at bedtime.

10. Apo-Cefaclor (cefaclor) suspension 250 milligrams by mouth three times each day.

11. Lasix (furosemide) 40 milligrams intravenously, immediately.

12. Heparin (heparin) 5 000 international units subcutaneously every morning and evening.

Systems of Measurement

OBJECTIVES

Système International d'Unités (SI)

The student will:

- identify the components of SI used in medication administration
- identify the rules associated with use of SI
- become familiar with the metric system and be able to:
  - state a definition of the metric system
  - identify the units of measurement within the metric system
  - identify the prefixes and symbols used in the metric system
  - correctly convert measurement amounts within the metric system
- become familiar with the use of moles and be able to:
  - state a definition of moles
  - identify the use of moles in medication administration
- become familiar with equivalents and be able to:
  - state a definition of equivalents
  - identify the use of equivalents in medication administration
- understand the concept of units and be able to:
  - state a definition of units
  - identify the use of units in medication administration

Apothecary System

The student will:

- state a definition of the apothecary system
- identify the use of the apothecary system in medication administration
- correctly carry out common conversions between the apothecary and metric systems

Household Measurement System

The student will:

- state a definition of the household measurement system
- identify the use of the household measurement system in medication administration
- correctly carry out common conversions between the household measurement and metric systems

24-Hour Clock

- The student will correctly make conversions between the 12-hour and 24-hour clocks

Système International (SI): the internationally agreed-upon system of measurement that is used by most of the countries of the world.

Metric system: decimal-based system of measurement that has been incorporated into Système International.

Moles: units of measurement of the amount of a substance; contain the same number of particles as there are atoms in 12 g of carbon-12.

Equivalent: the amount of a substance that would react with or replace 1 g of hydrogen.

International units (IU): internationally agreed-upon amount of a substance with a specific biological effect.

Apothecary system: old English system of measuring amounts of drugs.

Household system: measurement system based on utensils usually found in a patient's home.

24-hour clock: designation of time that begins 1 minute after midnight at 0001 hours and continues to midnight, or 2400 hours.

In a sense, all measurement systems are arbitrary, whether the basic unit is the length of the king's foot or the length of a sonar pulse. The important thing is to arrive at some standard understood and accepted by everyone. This is especially important in medicine, because physicians have to be able to order specific medications in specific quantities, knowing that the dosage units are universally understood.

In medical applications, the key measure is weight per unit of volume. This states the amount of medication in a given solid (tablet or capsule) or liquid (oral liquids or parenteral) form. If no common measurement system is in effect, the chance of errors in dosage is enormous.

Système International d'Unités (International System of Units) (SI)

Système International (SI) is the internationally agreed system of measurement used by most of the countries of the world, Canada included. SI has seven categories, each of which has a principal unit (Table 4.1).

Each of the principal units has a very specific definition. Prefixes are used to identify decimal fractions of each unit.

The categories used in the administration of medications are length, mass, and amount of substance. Volume is derived from length, and weight is derived from mass.

As well as medications, most diagnostic test results will be expressed in SI units. When evaluating diagnostic test results, you must make sure that the reference values are in SI units. (Note: Some reference books that originate in the United States do not use SI units.)

TABLE 4.1
CATEGORIES OF SI

Category	Principal Unit	Abbreviation
Length	metre	m
Mass	kilogram	kg
Time	second	s
Electric current	ampere	A
Temperature	kelvin	K
Amount of substance	mole	mol
Luminous intensity	candela	cd

Rules of SI Usage

A set of rules for using SI units has been identified.

1. Units are given one prefix only. Microgram is correct, millimilligram is not correct.
2. Prefixes that make a unit larger are written in uppercase letters (Mega, Giga), while prefixes that make a unit smaller are written in lowercase letters (centi, milli). The exception to this is kilo, which is written in lower case to avoid confusion with degrees Kelvin. When it stands alone, Litre is always capitalized (L) to avoid confusion between the number 1 and a lowercase l. Lowercase is used when it is part of a compound measure such as millilitre.
3. Abbreviations of units are *never* pluralized. 5 kilograms is abbreviated to 5 kg, not kgs.
4. An abbreviation is never followed by a period unless it occurs at the end of a sentence.
5. The numbers are separated from the units by a space: 2 ml is correct, 2ml is not.
6. Large numbers are made easier to read by inserting a space between groups of three numbers. Commas are not used to separate the groups of three. One million is written 1 000 000 not 1,000,000.
7. In English-speaking countries, decimal fractions are written with a period between the whole number and the fraction, e.g., 1.75. In Europe, a comma separates the whole

number from the fraction, e.g., 1,75. Quebec usually follows the English convention, but there is variation of usage in the rest of the world. When the period is used, care must be taken to place it on the line of the bottom edge of the numbers and not in the middle, where it might be confused with a hyphen or some other symbol.

Metric System

When the Système International was established in 1960, it included the metric system, which was developed in France in 1795. It established the standards for length, volume, and weight that we now use for medication administration.

The metric system is based on multiples of 10. Prefixes are attached to the base unit, and each prefix indicates by how many 10s the base unit is multiplied or divided (Table 4.2).

TABLE 4.2
SI UNITS

1 000	100	10	1	$\frac{1}{10}$	$\frac{1}{100}$	$\frac{1}{1\,000}$	$\frac{1}{1\,000\,000}$	$\frac{1}{1\,000\,000\,000}$
thousands	hundreds	tens	ones	tenths	hundredths	thousandths	millionths	billionths
kilo	Hecto	Deka		deci	centi	milli	micro	nano
k	H	Dk		d	c	m	mc μ	n
10^3	10^2	10^1		10^{-1}	10^{-2}	10^{-3}	10^{-6}	10^{-9}
1 000	100	10		0.1	0.01	0.001	0.000001	0.000000001
Units larger than the base unit have Greek prefixes				———— Units smaller than the base unit ———— have Latin prefixes				

When going from a smaller to a larger unit, e.g., milligrams to grams, the decimal point moves to the left: 500 mg = 0.5 g.

When moving from a larger to a smaller unit, e.g., Litres to millilitres, the decimal point moves to the right: 2 L = 2 000 ml.

MAKE A NOTE

When converting between micrograms (mcg or μg) and milligrams, the decimal point moves 3 places: mcg or μg to mg moves 3 places left, mg to mcg or μg moves 3 places right.

When converting between milligrams (mg) and grams (g), the decimal point also moves 3 places: mg to g moves 3 places to the left, g to mg moves 3 places right.

YOU TRY IT

(The answers to these questions are found at the end of the book.)

Convert the following values within the metric system.

1. 750 mg = _____ g

2. 2 L = _____ ml

3. 5 kg = _____ g

4. 1.5 g = _____ mg

5. 500 mg = _____ kg

6. 200 μg = _____ mg

The base unit for weight in the metric system is the gram. Drugs are usually ordered in grams or milligrams (one-thousandth of a gram), e.g., **Gravol (dimenhydrinate) 50 mg.**

The base unit for volume in the metric system is the litre. Drugs in liquid form are usually a solution that is identified by its concentration or the number of milligrams in each millilitre of fluid, e.g., *Gravol (dimenhydrinate) 50 mg/ml.*

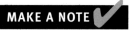

MAKE A NOTE ✔

Volume may also be stated in cubic centimetres. 1 cubic centimetre (cc) = 1 millilitre (ml). The terms may be used interchangeably.

Although most drugs are measured in milligrams per millilitre, or mg/ml, there are other systems that you may encounter in specific situations.

Moles

In the Système International, a mole is the standard unit to measure the amount of a substance. A mole of a substance is the amount containing the same number of elementary particles (atoms, molecules, ions, or other particles) as there are atoms in 12 g of carbon-12, which is 6.02×10^{23}. A mole of any substance is the molecular weight of that substance in grams. For example, potassium chloride (KCl) has a molecular weight of 74.5. (Potassium has an atomic weight of 39.09 and chlorine has an atomic weight of 35.45. There is one molecule of potassium and one molecule of chlorine in potassium chloride, so the molecular weight of KCl is 74.5). Thus the mole-to-gram relation for KCl is

$$1 \text{ mole KCl} = 74.5 \text{ g KCl.}$$

Moles are used primarily in chemistry, but there are a few drugs, usually electrolytes such as potassium chloride, that are ordered in moles. Moles are relatively large amounts, so the drug order is usually stated in millimoles: 1 mmol of KCl = 0.0745 g or 74.5 mg.

Equivalents

An equivalent weight is also a term primarily used in chemistry. It represents the amount of a substance that would react with or replace one gram of hydrogen. It is calculated by dividing the molecular weight by the valence of the molecule. As with moles, the amount is relatively large, so drug orders are usually stated in milliequivalents (mEq). The most common drugs ordered in milliequivalents are also electrolytes. The preparations are manufactured as mEq/ml, e.g., **KCl 20 mEq/ml.**

Units or International Units (IU)

Units are used to measure the activity of a given substance. For each substance that is measured in units, there is an international agreement specifying the biological effect expected with a dose of 1 IU, e.g., 1 unit of insulin lowers blood sugar by a specific amount.

The medications usually ordered in units, or IU, include insulin, heparin, penicillin, and most vitamins.

There is no definite conversion between IU and milligrams because different preparations vary in their biological activity. In other words, an mg of heparin manufactured in France may be more active than a mg of heparin manufactured in Canada, but the amounts are adjusted so that a unit of French heparin has the same biological effect as a unit of Canadian heparin. These preparations are manufactured as units or iu/ml, e.g., **heparin 5 000 iu/ml.**

Apothecary System

The apothecary system is the old English system of measuring amounts of drugs. It has been almost completely replaced by SI/metric in Canada. The unit of weight is the grain and the unit of volume is the dram. The conversion is not exact, which is one of the reasons that use of the apothecary system is discouraged.

1 grain (gr) = 60 or 65 mg

1 dram (ʒ) = 4 ml

To give you an idea of how antique this system is, quantity in the apothecary system is identified in Roman numerals, e.g., *ASA gr v* means *5 grains of ASA (acetylsalicylic acid)*.

This is the only element of the apothecary system that still lingers in current usage. Some physicians still write the number of tablets to be given in Roman numerals, e.g., Tylenol 300 mg tabs ii. This means that you will give two 300 mg tablets, or 600 mg.

Household System

The household system of measurement was based on the utensils that a physician might reasonably expect to find in the patient's home, back when doctors made house calls. It is rarely used now other than for prescription of oral liquids, usually for children. The household measures that are helpful to know are

1 teaspoon (t, tsp, teas) = 5 ml

1 tablespoon (T, Tb, Tbs) = 15 ml

1 ounce (oz) = 30 ml

Liquid medication delivery devices such as droppers and spoons (Figure 4-1) are now readily available from most pharmacies at reasonable cost, so the use of the household system is gradually declining.

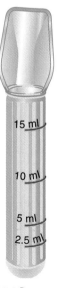

FIGURE 4-1 Dosage spoon.

24-Hour Clock

The traditional 12-hour clock uses the designations AM and PM to indicate morning or afternoon. This may cause confusion if the designations are not clearly written. To avoid this problem, hospitals and other health care settings in Canada use the 24-hour clock.

The 24-hour clock begins at 0001 hours, or 1 minute after midnight, and runs for 24 hours to 2400 hours, or midnight; AM and PM are omitted, as is the colon that usually separates hours from minutes. The hours from 0 to 9 are preceded by a 0. The times from 0001 to 1259 are essentially the same as the 12-hour clock. Starting at 1 PM, 12 is added to the hours until midnight. For example,

1 am = 0100 hr

1:30 am = 0130 hr

6:45 am = 0645

11:15 am = 1115 hrs

1 pm = 1300 hrs

1:30 pm = 1330 hrs

6:45 pm = 1845 hrs

11:15 pm = 2315 hrs

Figures 4-2 and 4-3 show examples of 12-hour and 24-hour clocks.

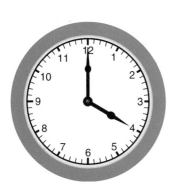

FIGURE 4-2 12-hour clock showing 4:00. This may be 4:00 PM or 4:00 AM.

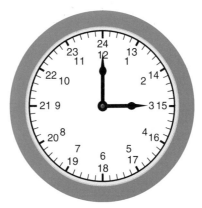

FIGURE 4-3 24-hour clock showing 1500 hrs or 3:00 PM.

YOU TRY IT

(The answers to these questions are found at the end of the book.)

Convert these 12-hour clock times to 24-hour clock times.

1. 4 PM _____

2. 3:15 AM _____

3. 2:45 AM _____

4. 11:40 PM _____

5. 11:40 AM _____

Convert these 24-hour clock times to 12-hour clock times.

6. 0430 _____

7. 1545 _____

8. 1910 _____

9. 0800 _____

10. 1240 _____

chapter 4

Self Test

Answers to these questions are found at the end of the book.

Identify which of the following are correct according to the rules of SI usage. For those that are not, write the correct form in the following space.

1. Centigram _____

2. 1,000,000 _____

3. 10 mg _____

4. 15 kg _____

5. 25 l _____

Change the following amounts from grams (g) to milligrams (mg).

6. 0.05 g _____ mg

7. 2.3 g _____ mg

8. 0.4 g _____ mg

9. 1.2 g _____ mg

10. 0.006 g _____ mg

Change the following amounts from milligrams (mg) to grams (g).

11. 25 mg _____ g

12. 200 mg _____ g

13. 1 mg _____ g

14. 1200 mg _____ g

15. 500 mg _____ g

Change the following amounts from micrograms (mcg or µg) to milligrams (mg).

16. 1 mcg _____ mg

17. 250 µg _____ mg

18. 100 µg _____ mg

19. 40 mcg _____ mg

20. 600 μg _____ mg

Change the following amounts from milligrams (mg) to micrograms (mcg or μg).

21. 1 mg _____ μg

22. 0.005 mg _____ mcg

23. 0.0007 mg _____ mcg

24. 20 mg _____ μg

25. 0.025 mg _____ mcg

Multiple Choice Questions

26. A mole is a measurement of which of the following?
    A. The amount of a substance that will combine with 1 g of hydrogen.
    B. An internationally agreed-upon amount that has a specific biological effect.
    C. The amount of a substance that contains the same number of particles as there are atoms in 12 g of carbon-12.
    D. The unit of weight in the apothecary system.

27. A grain is a measurement of which of the following?
    A. The amount of a substance that will combine with 1 g of hydrogen.
    B. An internationally agreed-upon amount that has a specific biological effect.
    C. The amount of a substance that contains the same number of particles as there are atoms in 12 g of carbon-12.
    D. The unit of weight in the apothecary system.

28. A unit is a measurement of which of the following?
    A. The amount of a substance that will combine with 1 g of hydrogen.
    B. An internationally agreed-upon amount that has a specific biological effect.
    C. The amount of a substance that contains the same number of particles as there are atoms in 12 g of carbon-12.
    D. The unit of weight in the apothecary system.

29. An equivalent is a measurement of which of the following?
    A. The amount of a substance that will combine with 1 g of hydrogen.
    B. An internationally agreed-upon amount that has a specific biological effect.
    C. The amount of a substance that contains the same number of particles as there are atoms in 12 g of carbon-12.
    D. The unit of weight in the apothecary system.

30. It is after noon and you check your watch to discover the time. Identify the 24-hour clock time for each of the watch faces below.

30a.

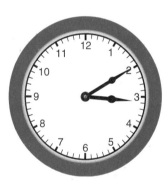

30b.

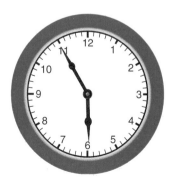

30c.

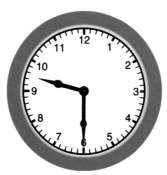

30d.

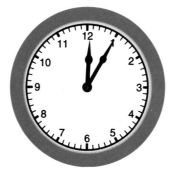

30e.

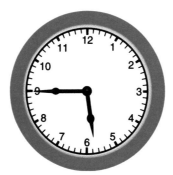

Components of a Doctor's Order

The student will:

- identify the components of a doctor's order
- identify the two classification systems for drugs
- know the conventions for the nomenclature of drugs
- identify the routes by which medications are given
- identify the various preparations used in medication routes
- interpret the frequency with which the medication should be given

Doctor's order: written or verbal directions from a physician or other qualified health professional; provides necessary authorization for the administration of medications.

Drug classifications: systems of organizing medications into categories. There are two classification systems: **functional class**—based on the physiological effect that the drug is designed to produce (e.g., antianginal drugs prevent or decrease angina); and **chemical class**—based on the biological action of the drug (e.g., H-2 receptor antagonists block the stimulation of H-2 receptors by histamine).

Generic drug name: name given to a drug when it is licensed. Each drug has only one generic name.

Trade drug name: name given to a drug by the individual manufacturer. A drug may have at least as many trade names as it does manufacturers.

Components of a Doctor's Order

In the institutional setting, medications are administered in accordance with an order written by a qualified health professional. Legislation varies somewhat from province to province, but orders may be written by dentists, optometrists, nurse practitioners, and midwives as well as physicians. These health practitioners are allowed to write certain types of orders under certain circumstances. Since these orders are usually called *doctor's orders*, this designation will be used for orders written by any qualified health professional (Figure 5-1).

The order is usually written on the doctor's order sheet in the patient's chart. To be legal, the order must contain the following information:

- Date the order is written. If the start date is different from the date the order is written, this date must be included as well.
- Full name of the patient
- Name of the drug
- Dose
- Route
- The frequency with which it is to be given
- Physician's signature

A physician may give a verbal or telephone order that is transcribed by a registered nurse, but the order must be signed by the physician within a given period of time (usually 24 hours).

AGH	4139702
Anywhere General Hospital	Allenby, Frederic
	1914 Dundas St.
	Apt 204
	Anywhere, Ontario

Doctor's Orders

Date	Orders
07/04/04	Digoxin 0.25 mg po OD
	furosemide 40 mg po bid
	ntg sray tt prn for chest pain
	repeat x 2 q 10 min if unrelieved
	morphine 10 mg sc if ntg not effective
	Ativan 0.5 mg sl q4h prn
	Zantac 150 mg po bid
	Enalapril 10 mg po bid
	Lee Chan MD

FIGURE 5-1 Doctor's orders.

Patient

Almost all the medication orders are written for specific patients. An order is written in an individual patient's chart, or a prescription is written for a specific person. There are two exceptions to this:

1. In some settings, where the patient problems are highly predictable, there may be preprinted order sheets (Figure 5-2). Some physicians almost always leave these orders as is; others cross out or change some of the orders, leaving most of them intact. The physician must write or stamp the patient's name on the sheet and sign it before the orders can be carried out.

2. The second exception is the standing order, or medical directive. In this case, the Medical Advisory Committee for the institution establishes a policy for giving certain medications without a specific order in a restricted set of circumstances. One of the commonest standing orders is for acetaminophen. The policy might state

AGH
Anywhere General Hospital

4587392
Donne, Susan
123 Main St.
Anywhere, Ontario

STANDARD ADMISSION ORDERS
MEDICINE
INSTRUCTIONS:
Strike out orders that are not applicable

Date _June 30, 2004_   Time _0400 hrs_
DIAGNOSIS _COPD, Pneumonia_

1. Admit to Dr. _Grant_ for primary care.   2. Telemetry   Yes ☐   No ☑

3. Diet as tolerated ☑ or_____   4. Activity as tolerated ☐ or _BRP_

5. IV: _2/3 + 1/3_ TKVO or _____   6. Vital Signs: BID or _TID_

7. O2 by nasal cannula at 3 L/min or _____

8. PRN Medications: (Strike out orders that are not applicable)
    Acetaminophen 650 mg po q4h prn
    ~~Dimenhydrinate 50 mg po, IM, IV q4h prn~~
    Docusate sodium 100 mg po tid prn
    Magnesium aluminum hydroxide gel 30 mL po q4h prn
    Oxazepam 10–15 mg po qhs prn

9. Routine Medications, Lab, Radiology, Treatments
    Solumedrol 80 mg IV qid
    Ancef 1 gram IV q6h
    Ventolin 1 mL c̄ Atrovent 2 mL by nebulizer q4h
    Chest X-ray
    CBC and lytes
    Physio consult in am

Mary Stevenson MD
Physician's Signature

FIGURE 5-2 Preprinted order sheet.

that a nurse may give acetaminophen for fever. The policy will define the specific circumstances (e.g., temperature greater than 38.5°C) and the dose (e.g., 650 mg). Medications covered by standing orders may not be given for any reason other than that stated in the order, e.g., the order cannot be used to administer acetaminophen for pain. The policy also defines the circumstances under which the nurse must notify the doctor that the policy has been implemented. This is usually within the next 12 or 24 hours. When administering medications by standing order, you must chart the problem and the action taken, e.g., "Temperature 39.3°C. Acetaminophen 650 mg PO given per standing order 4.12.3."

CRITICAL THINKING

You are caring for Maggie Fraser, a 27-year-old woman who has had multiple admissions to your unit. She tells you that she usually takes 50 mg of dimenhydrinate each night to sleep and asks you to bring her some. You tell her that the doctor has not ordered any for her. She tells you that she knows that your hospital has a standing order for dimenhydrinate. You tell her that the order states that the dimenhydrinate is to be given only for nausea.

Twenty minutes later, she calls and tells you that she is nauseated and needs some dimenhydrinate.

What should be your response to this request?

Drug

A drug is a chemical substance that modifies physiological function. It may:

- replace a body function, e.g., insulin
- enhance or increase a body function, e.g., salbutamol increases bronchodilation
- impede or decrease a function, e.g., morphine decreases the transmission of pain impulses
- destroy unwanted tissue, e.g., antineoplastics destroy cancer cells
- destroy or neutralize substances from outside the body, e.g., antibiotics

Drug Classifications

Drugs are categorized by both functional class and by chemical class.

The **functional class** of a drug is based on the physiological effect that the drug is designed to produce. Antihypertensives are a functional class of drugs that lower blood pressure.

The **chemical class** is based on the biological action of the drug. Beta (β) blockers are drugs that block the action of adrenalin on beta-adrenergic receptors.

Functional classes may contain a number of different chemical classes. Antihypertensives include β blockers, calcium channel blockers, ACE inhibitors and thiazide diuretics. A drug in one chemical class may belong in a number of different functional classes. β blockers act as antihypertensives, antiarrhythmics and antianginals.

It is important to know the classes of drugs. Knowing the functional class allows you to anticipate and evaluate the effect of the drug. Knowing the chemical class gives you an indication of adverse effects that might occur as a result of the drug.

Finding out about drug classifications, usual doses, effects, side effects, and nursing responsibilities can be done with one of the many drug handbooks available for sale. It is good practice to own a handbook and keep it with you when you are preparing medications. Note that there are presently no Canadian handbooks—those widely available are published in the United States. This means that some drugs are not listed in the handbooks, while others are not identified by their Canadian trade names.

If you cannot find a drug in your handbook, check the *Compendium of Pharmaceuticals and Specialties (CPS)*. There is usually a copy of it on hospital units or in the hospital pharmacy. Published by the Canadian Pharmacies Association, this book covers all drugs sold in Canada and contains product monographs for most drugs. It generally contains information about the drug classification, the pharmacokinetics and pharmacodynamics of the drug, the usual dose, and how the drug is supplied. It does not cover nursing responsibilities, so don't use the *CPS* as your primary source of information.

If all else fails, your final resort is to call the pharmacist who dispensed the drug. Most of them are very happy to share their information with you.

Drug Nomenclature

A fruitful source of errors in administration of medications is the thorny tangle of names applied to drugs. Each drug gets an official, or generic, name when it's originally licensed, e.g., *diazepam*. Then each manufacturer gives the drug a brand, *proprietary*, name: *Valium, Epam, Vivol, etc.* You can tell them apart because the generic name usually starts with a lower-case letter, while the brand name has a capital letter.

In the clinical setting, nomenclature is inconsistent. Some doctors order some drugs by their generic names, e.g., *codeine*; other times an order will use the brand name, e.g., *Pyridium*. If this isn't confusing enough, with some drugs the generic name and the brand name are used interchangeably, e.g., *Lasix/furosemide*.

Some of the examples in this book will identify drugs by their generic name, some by their proprietary name, and some by both—just like the real world.

Dose

The dose is the amount of the drug to be given. In most cases, this is the weight of the drug measured in milligrams.

Drugs come in various forms. The solid forms are tablets, sublingual solids, suppositories, and transdermal patches. Their dosage is calculated in weight per unit: milligrams per tablet or milligrams per patch.

If a drug is manufactured in only one dosage, the physician might order it by the number of units, e.g., *Gravol 1 tablet q4h prn*. This happens most often with a tablet that contains more than one drug, such as Arthrotec 50—it contains 50 mg of diclofenac and 200 mEq of misoprostol. An order might be written as *Arthrotec tabs i bid*.

You'll occasionally see an order with the drug, the dose, and the number of tablets all stated, e.g., *Isoptin 120 mg tabs ii bid*. This means the physician wants the patient to have two tablets, each containing 120 mg of a drug (i.e., 240 mg) twice a day. Most hospitals discourage this type of order, but some physicians are set in their ways and resist changing their habits.

Drugs that come in liquid form are usually solutions with a given weight of the drug per unit of volume. The doctor's order will state the weight of the drug to be given, while the package in which the drug comes will identify the strength of the solution. For example, the physician will order furosemide as *Lasix 20 mg IV*. The package will show the strength of the solution as 10 mg/ml. (See Chapter 8 for the methodology used to calculate the number of millilitres to give.)

Route

There are three major ways, or *routes*, by which a drug can be given: oral, parenteral, and topical. Oral drugs are taken into the mouth and swallowed, being absorbed through the gastrointestinal mucosa into the body. Parenteral drugs are those that enter the body by any means other than the gastric mucosa; both oral and parenteral drugs have systemic effects. Topical medications are applied to either the skin or the mucous membrane and have a local effect; they're not absorbed into the body and do not have a systemic effect. Within each category, there is a variety of preparations.

Oral Medications

Oral Liquids

These are intended to be swallowed and are usually the most quickly absorbed from the GI tract.

- *Aqueous solutions* have one or more drugs dissolved in water.
- *Aqueous suspensions* have one or more drugs finely divided and mixed with water. These appear opaque or cloudy. The particles settle on the bottom of the container, so you have to shake the mixture before pouring it.
- *Fluid extract* is a concentrated drug mixed with alcohol. It is the most concentrated of all liquid preparations.
- *Elixir* is a drug mixed with a sweetened and aromatic solution of alcohol.
- *Syrup* is a drug mixed with water and sugar to disguise an unpleasant taste.

Oral Solids

These drugs are mixed with inert material to form a small solid object that is intended to be swallowed.

- *Tablets* are powdered drugs mixed with an inert substance and compressed into small hard discs (Figure 5-3). Some tablets are scored so that they can be cut into fractions, and most tablets can be crushed for patients who are unable to swallow them.

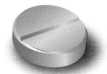

FIGURE 5-3 Tablet.

- *Caplets* are tablets formed into an oblong shape. Some of them have a gelatin coating to make them easier to swallow.
- *Capsules* have powdered medication encased in a two-part gelatin coating (Figure 5-4). With some capsules, the coating can be taken apart and the powdered medication mixed with food or water.

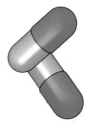

FIGURE 5-4 Capsules.

- *Enteric-coated* (EC) *tablets* have a protective coating that is resistant to stomach acids. That makes them dissolve in the duodenum, not the stomach, in order to protect the GI tract from irritation. EC tablets should not be crushed or broken, because that defeats the purpose of the coating.

Parenteral Medications

Parenteral medications are those that enter the body by some means other than the GI tract. This category includes drugs absorbed through mucous membranes or through the skin, as well as those that are injected.

Mucous Membrane Medications

- *Sublingual medications* are tiny, concentrated tablets that dissolve quickly when placed under the tongue. The medication is absorbed through the oral mucous membrane directly into the bloodstream.

- *Buccal medications* are placed in the cheek or chewed slowly so the drug can be absorbed through the oral mucous membrane.
- *Inhaled medications* usually act directly on receptors in the mucous membrane to give a systemic effect but are not absorbed into the bloodstream.
  - *Metered dose inhalers* (puffers), shown in Figure 5-5, are pressurized sprays that deliver medication directly to the nose or lungs.
  - *Nebulizers* (Figure 5-6) deliver a medicated mist that can be inhaled. Compressed air is forced into a liquid medication, turning the liquid into a mist.

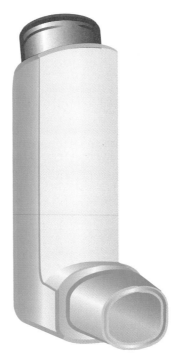

FIGURE 5-5 Metered dose inhaler.

- *Rectal* medication is placed against the mucous membrane of the rectum for absorption into the bloodstream.
  - *Suppositories* (Figure 5-7) are semisolids in which the medication is mixed with a base such as gelatin and shaped for insertion into the body. The base gradually dissolves at body temperature and the medication is slowly absorbed through the mucosa, releasing it into the bloodstream.
  - *Enemas* contain a medication in liquid form. The diluted drug is instilled into the rectum where it can act locally or be absorbed.

Transdermal Medications

Transdermal medications are applied to the skin to be absorbed into the vascular system. Absorption is much slower than through mucous membranes. These medications are generally used to provide a small but continuous supply of drug so that there is very little variation in serum drug levels. Most transdermal medications are in the form of self–adhesive patches that are left in place for up to 72 hours.

Injectable Medications

A needle is used to pierce the skin and deliver the medication to the appropriate body tissue.

- *Subdermal* medication is injected just under the dermal layer. This route is usually used only for diagnostic testing.
- *Subcutaneous (SC)* medication is injected into the subcutaneous layer. It has the slowest absorption rate of the usual parenteral routes.

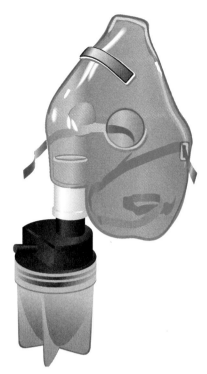

FIGURE 5-6 Nebulizer.

FIGURE 5-7 Suppository.

- *Intramuscular (IM)* medication is injected into a muscle. It is absorbed more quickly than SC, but the patient usually finds it more painful.
- *Intravenous (IV)* medication is injected or infused directly into a vein. Of the usual injectable routes, IV acts the most quickly.
- *Intracardiac* medication can be injected directly into the heart muscle. This is usually only done by a physician during treatment of a cardiac arrest.
- *Intrathecal* medication is injected into the subdural space of the spinal cord. It is infrequently used and may be carried out by physicians only.

Topical Medications

Topical medications are those that are applied to skin or mucous membrane for local effect only.

- *Troches, lozenges,* and *pastilles* are preparations that dissolve in the mouth and are usually designed to treat topical conditions of the mouth and oropharynx.
- *Creams, lotions, ointments, liniments*, and *pastes* contain medication to treat skin disorders on contact.
- *Ophthalmic medications* are preparations used to treat disorders of the eye.
  - *Drops* and *creams* can be inserted into the eye to treat local disorders or alter the functioning of the eye.
  - *Intraocular disks* are similar to a contact lens and are inserted into the patient's eye. They contain a drug that is absorbed into the aqueous humor over a specific period of time.
- *Otic medications* are drops inserted into the ear to treat local infections or decrease pain.

- *Rectal suppositories* and *enemas* may be intended to act locally rather than be absorbed.
- *Vaginal medications* are usually used to treat local infections or inflammatory disorders.

Frequency

The doctor's order must also include the frequency with which the drug is given. The physician may state the number of times per day a drug is given, e.g., BID or QID, or identify the number of hours between doses, e.g., q4h or q6h. (See Chapter 3 for abbreviations.)

Once the doctor has identified the frequency, agency policy usually determines the actual time at which the medication should be given, e.g., QID medications may be given at 0800, 1200, 1600, and 2200. The intervals between these medications are not necessarily equal, although they are usually spread out between the normal hours of waking and sleeping. When it is pharmacologically necessary, the physician may order the medication to be given at specific times of the day, e.g., AC or HS.

When the order calls for a specific interval between doses, an agency may identify standard times, e.g., medications ordered q6h may be routinely given at 0600, 1200, 1800, and 2400 hours. In other places, the first dose may be given as soon as the drug is ordered; subsequent doses follow at the appropriate interval.

Some medications are to be given only if they're needed. They're ordered the same way as any other drug, except they're identified as PRN on the order sheet. Sometimes the doctor will include the circumstances under which the medication is to be given, e.g., *Gravol (dimenhydrinate) 50 mg IM for nausea PRN*. Other doctors will assume the nurse has enough knowledge and judgment to administer the medication appropriately.

Self Test

Answers to these questions are found at the end of the book.

1. Which of the following doctor's orders must be signed by the physician?
   A. Preprinted order sheets
   B. Standing orders
   C. Telephone orders
   D. All doctor's orders

2. Identify which of the following represent a functional classification and which of the following represent a chemical classification:
   A. β blockers
   B. Antihypertensives
   C. Antianginals
   D. ACE inhibitors

3. Which of the following liquid medications contain alcohol?
   A. Elixir
   B. Aqueous suspension
   C. Syrup
   D. Fluid extract
   E. Aqueous solution

4. Enteric-coated tablets are designed to dissolve in which of the following parts of the GI tract?
   A. Esophagus
   B. Stomach
   C. Duodenum
   D. Jejunum

5. Your patient has an order for *morphine 5 mg any route q2h prn.* She states that she is having severe pain. You feel that it is important that she get relief from her pain as quickly as possible. Which of the following routes will you choose?
   A. Intravenous
   B. Intramuscular
   C. Subcutaneous
   D. Oral

6. Your patient has an order for *Maxeran (metoclopramide) 10 mg po qid AC and HS.* When will you give this drug?

7. Identify the omissions in the doctor's orders that are shown below.

AGH	5239802
Anywhere General Hospital	Boroski, George 178 Dufferin St. Anywhere, Ontario

Doctor's Orders

Date	Orders
19/06/04	celecoxib 200 mg bid
	Ventolin 2 puffs
	Prednisone 60 mg po qam
	Zinacef IV q8h
	Laxative of choice

Interpreting Drug Labels

OBJECTIVES

The student will:

- define and describe the components of a drug label
- correctly interpret the information on a drug label
  - manufacturer's label
  - hospital pharmacy label
  - unit dose label
  - pharmacist's label

KEY TERMS

Unit dose packaging: the hospital pharmacy individually packages each dose of a drug.

Over-the-counter (OTC) medications: drugs that can be purchased without a written prescription from a physician.

Prescription medications: These are drugs which require a prescription from a physician or other member of a Health Profession licensed to write a prescription for that drug.

Manufacturer's Label

Once you have interpreted the doctor's order, you will know the patient, the name of the drug, the dose, the route, and the time it is to be given. The next step is to get the right amount of the right drug from the container in which it is stored. You must be able to read and interpret the label on the container so that you can calculate how much of the drug you are going to give.

In the hospital setting, medications are usually in either the manufacturer's containers or containers prepared by the hospital pharmacy. The hospital pharmacy may prepare individual bottles of medication for each patient or unit dose packages. In community settings, the medications may be in containers from a commercial pharmacy.

Unfortunately, there is no consistency in how containers of drugs are labeled, and you need to take extra care to ensure you're interpreting the data correctly (Figure 6-1). There is considerable variation in style of manufacturers' labels, but they all contain much the same information. The label shown in Figure 6-1 is fairly typical.

Trade Name

Each manufacturer gives its own name to a drug and uses this *trade,* or copyrighted, name in its advertising. A drug manufactured by several different companies will have several different trade names.

Number of Units of Medication in Package

This tells you how many individual units of drug are in the package. For oral solids, this is the number of tablets, capsules, etc. Drugs in liquid form may be one single-use ampoule or a package containing a number of single-use ampoules. Liquid drugs may also be packaged as one unit or one or more multi-use vials.

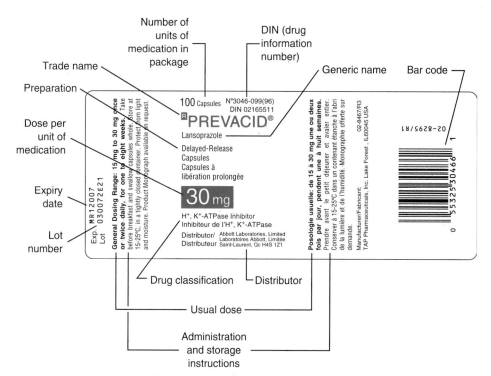

FIGURE 6-1 Manufacturer's label.

DIN (Drug Information Number)

Health Canada assigns this code to identify the drug. If you are looking for information about a drug on the Health Canada website, you must use this number to do your search.

Generic Name

This is the name given to a drug when it is licensed. This name is usually printed in smaller type than the trade name.

Bar Code

Retail stores use bar codes to identify products for price scanning and inventory control.

Manufacturer

This is the company that actually makes the drugs. In Canada, many large pharmaceutical companies subcontract the manufacturing to smaller companies.

Distributor

This is the company that advertises, markets, and sells the drug.

Usual Dose

This is the amount of medication normally ordered for a patient, usually one to two times the unit dose. In some cases, the physician may decide to go outside the usual dosage range in treating patients. When this occurs, it is important that the nurse know the reason for the change to help distinguish a treatment decision from an error by the physician.

Administration and Storage Instructions

A variety of information may be included on the package. You may find such details as instructions on mixing solutions, whether or not the drug should be taken with food, precautions about adverse effects, and whether tablets can be broken or crushed. Storage instructions might tell you whether the drug is to be refrigerated and if it should be kept out of direct sunlight.

Drug Classification

Some labels include the drug classification and may indicate the chemical or the functional class.

Lot Number

The manufacturers assign this number and use it to identify when and where the drug was produced. They need this in case of a problem with the manufacturing process that necessitates a recall.

Expiry Date

This is the date after which the drug should no longer be taken. This is not just a "best-before" date, and it is important to check the expiry date because some drugs lose their efficacy after this date, while others, such as tetracycline, become toxic as they age.

Dose per Unit of Medication

This is the strength of the medication. It is one of the key factors used to calculate the amount of drug to be given to the patient.

KEEP IT SAFE It is critical to identify the strength of the medication carefully, especially with liquid medications. Because there is no uniformity in labeling, the strength may be indicated in different ways. One drug may indicate the strength as 100 mg/5ml, another may indicate it as 20 mg/ml. For example, the label may read furosemide 40 mg, and elsewhere on the package, it may indicate that there are 4 ml in the ampoule. Be careful of labels that do not identify the strength at all. The package may merely state the number of millilitres and the number of milligrams in the package itself, and further calculations are up to the nurse.

Preparation

The type of preparation is important in administering the drug. Some oral solids may be crushed or halved; others may not—important information you need to consider in preparing the medication. (See Chapter 10 for information on the types of oral solids that can be crushed.)

Hospital Pharmacy Label

The information on the hospital pharmacy label (Figure 6-2) is much more patient-specific than the manufacturer's label. This information usually includes some or all of the following information.

Pharmacy Order Number

Hospital pharmacies usually assign some sort of number to track medication orders.

Generic Drug Name

Hospital pharmacies generally manage medications by generic name. Some institutions use only the generic name, while others include the trade name used by the physician when he ordered the drug. Still others identify all of the trade names under which that drug might be ordered.

KEEP IT SAFE The lack of consistency in the use of trade and generic drug names is a problem for most of us when we are pouring medications. Keep a drug guide with you while you are preparing your medications so that you can cross-check trade and generic names easily. (See Chapter 5 for information about drug guides.)

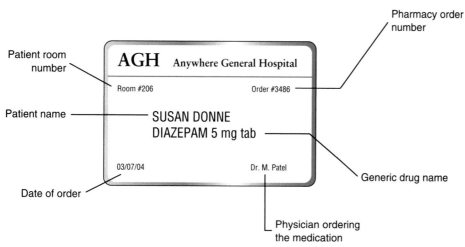

FIGURE 6-2 Hospital pharmacy label.

Physician Ordering the Medication

Most hospital pharmacies identify the physician who wrote the order on the label. This is helpful in verifying the doctor's order if any questions arise.

Date of the Order

Many institutions have automatic stop dates on some or all medication orders. Antibiotics and narcotic analgesics are most commonly given for limited periods of time before they must be reordered.

Patient Name and Room Number

Individual packages of medication are usually supplied for a specific patient. The dose for a specific patient should be taken from his or her individual package, even though you may have several patients on the same drug at the same time. Some institutions are very rigid about this; others are more relaxed and allow you to "borrow" medications from other patients' packages. Check the practice in your institution before borrowing.

Unit Dose Packaging

Unit dose packaging information tends to be minimal (Figure 6-3). It typically includes the name of the drug, usually only the generic name, and the dose included in the package. Sometimes the packages will be made up with a single tablet or capsule in them so you will still need to calculate the amount to be given using the methods outlined in Chapter 8.

Other institutions will prepare packages to match the doctor's order. If the order calls for two tablets or one-half tablet, the package will contain that amount and it will be noted on the label (Figure 6-4). Although this requires less calculation, it is still important to check the amount to ensure that the pharmacy has not made an error.

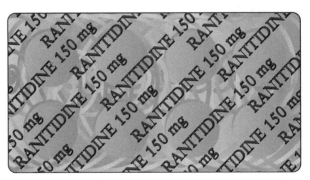

FIGURE 6-3 Unit dose package.

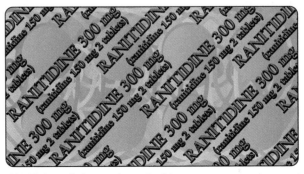

FIGURE 6-4 Unit dose package, 2 tablets.

Pharmacy Label

In community settings, patients usually purchase their medication from a commercial pharmacy. Most patients will have a combination of over-the-counter (OTC) medications and prescription medications. OTC medications will have a manufacturer's label on them. Prescription medications will have a label similar to the one in Figure 6-5 and tend to have more patient education information on them than do manufacturer's labels.

One of the roles of the community nurse is to assist patients in managing all of their medications. This usually includes patient teaching and may also include preparing medications on a daily or weekly basis. There are a variety of boxes or trays with individual compartments available for organizing patients' medications.

Patient Name

Pharmacy prescription labels always include the name of the patient for whom the medications is intended.

Directions for Taking Medication

These directions are usually written out in full and do not include the usual abbreviations seen in medical communications.

Number of Times Prescription Can Be Refilled

One of the responsibilities of the community nurse may be to monitor the amount of medication the patient has and to makes sure the supply is continually available. This number lets you know how soon the patient needs to visit the physician to have the medication reordered.

Date Prescription Was Filled

This date needs to be monitored to ensure that outdated medication does not pose a risk to the patient. If you are unsure of how long the medication remains good, the pharmacy that filled the prescription will be able to tell you.

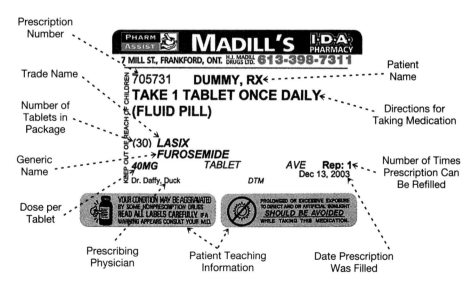

FIGURE 6-5 Pharmacy label.

Information for the Patient

Each of the provincial bodies overseeing the regulation of pharmacy and pharmacists is a member of the National Association of Pharmacy Regulatory Authorities (NAPRA). NAPRA makes recommendations for standards of practice, which become part of the regulatory bodies' provincial standards. The NAPRA Competency # 2 states that pharmacists shall provide drug information to their clients. This information is usually included on the labels of prescription drugs, but many pharmacies also give the patients printed drug information with their prescriptions. If your patient has some of these information sheets, they should be used as part of the teaching you are carrying out.

Prescribing Physician

Any questions or requests for refills of the medications should be directed to this physician. Should you need his address or phone number, the pharmacy will have it in their records.

Dose per Tablet

This is the strength of the medication. Along with the dosage instructions, this can be used to calculate how much medication your patient is taking.

Generic Name/Trade Name

Most pharmacies identify the trade name under which the drug was ordered, as well as the generic name of the drug.

Prescription Number

This number is used by the pharmacy to identify the individual prescription. This number should be given to the pharmacist when reordering the medication.

Self Test

Answers to these questions are found at the end of the book.

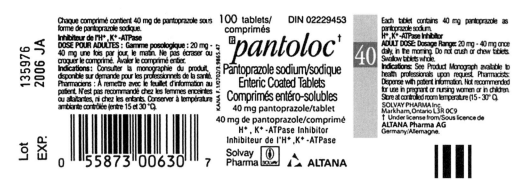

1. What is the generic name of this drug?

2. What is the adult dosage range?

3. What is the strength of the tablets?

4. What is the expiry date?

5. Who should not take this drug?

6. Who manufactured this drug?

7. What preparation are these tablets?

8. Where should these tablets be stored?

9. What is the lot number of this package?

10. What class of drug is this?

Medication Systems

OBJECTIVES

The student will:

■ **identify the components of a Medication Administration Record (MAR)**
■ **describe the following medication delivery systems:**
  - **unit dose**
  - **individual bottles**
  - **stock supply**
  - **computerized systems**

KEY TERMS

MAR (Medication Administration Record): the hospital document upon which is recorded the drug, dose, route, and time that medications are to be administered. It is signed by the nurse to indicate that the medication has been given.

Medication Administration Record

Once the doctor has written an order for a medication, the order is copied to a Medication Administration Record (MAR). This may be done by a nurse or a ward secretary. Hospital policy defines who is responsible for copying orders and who may check that they are accurate. Computerized systems may create the MAR when the original order is entered into the computer. The information on the MAR includes the following:

- Name of the patient
- Any medication allergies
- Drug name
- Dose
- Route
- Frequency
- Any special instruction

Sign the MAR in the space provided as soon as you have given each patient the medication. It is not safe to wait until medications have been given to a group of patients before you sign for all of them.

Many settings use separate MARs for regular and PRN medications. Other settings use the front side of the sheet for regular medications and the back for PRNs. Stat medications may have a separate sheet, or a designated area on the regular or PRN sheet (Figures 7-1 and 7-2).

KEEP IT SAFE The MAR also ensures that you give the right drug to the right patient. You should take the MAR to the bedside with the medication and compare it to the patient's arm band to decrease the chance of errors.

A requisition is usually sent to the hospital pharmacy when the order is transferred. The pharmacy then ensures that there is a supply of the drug available for the nurse to administer. There are a variety of systems for supplying the drugs to a hospital unit.

Medication Delivery Systems

In a hospital, as in any large institution, there are systems or procedures or protocols set up to ensure certain things are done in certain ways. A hotel will have a schedule for collecting, sorting, and cleaning linen, for example, because guests expect neatly made beds.

In a medical setting, one of the important things to do is to deliver and administer medications. That's why there are procedures set up for doing this. The underlying idea is to give you a set of routines that you can learn and follow. But given the importance of medication, it's essential that you follow the procedures intelligently, not blindly. Different institutions employ different systems for the delivery of medications.

Unit Dose Systems

With a unit dose system, the patients' medications are delivered on a daily basis. There is usually a cart that contains a drawer for each patient on each unit. The pharmacy, with the medication orders on hand, is responsible for filling up each drawer with the right medications. Please note: this doesn't mean the nurse has no responsibility—we'll discuss that later. A 24-hour supply of medication is prepared by the hospital pharmacy and delivered to the hospital unit every day.

In preparing the drawer for the orders noted on the MAR in Figure 7-1, the pharmacy would put in the following: one package each of glyburide 5 mg and glyburide 2.5 mg; one package of Pravachol 40 mg; two packages of Cardizem SR 90 mg; and three

Init	Signature
RS	R Spear RN
AB	A Barri RPN
LO'H	LO'Hara RN

AGH
Anywhere General Hospital
MEDICATION
ADMINISTRATION
RECORD

4476392
Desmarais, Pierre
144 King St.
Anywhere,
Ontario

Allergies	Penicillin sulfonamides

Diagnosis	Diabetes, PVD, cellulitis

Scheduled Medication	Time	June 10	June 11	June 12	June 13	June 14	June 15	June 16	June 17
glyburide 5 mg po- pc breakfast	0800	RS	RS						
glyburide 2.5 mg po- pc supper	1700	RS	RS						
Cardizem SR 90 mg po BID	0800	RS	RS						
	1800	RS							
Ancef 1 g IV Q8H	0600	LO'H	LO'H						
	1400	RS	RS						
	2200	LO'H							
Pravachol 40 mg po QHS	2200	AB							

FIGURE 7-1 MAR for regular medications.

packages of Ancef 1 g. Note that Ancef may come in the form of a vial—meaning it has to be mixed and added to a soluset or minibag—or it may come premixed. (That's what we mean by using the system intelligently.)

In the drawer holding the medications ordered in the MAR in Figure 7-2, there would be one package each of Dulcolax 5 mg for oral use and one Dulcolax 5 mg suppository. The Tylenol # 3 and lorazepam won't be in the drawer; you'll find them in the narcotics cupboard, because they're both drugs that fall under the Controlled Drugs and Substances Act. (More about this cupboard later.)

Many people consider the unit dose system to be safer than some of the alternatives, because only the drugs applicable to an individual patient are in the patient's drawer. Being an intelligent user of the system, of course, you'll know that it's still vital for you to check the name and dose against the MAR as you would with any other system.

Individual Containers

Some institutions use a system in which the pharmacy prepares a bottle or package of medication for each patient, according to the order. The container should give the name and room number of the patient. With this system, filling the orders in

Init	Signature
RS	R Spear RN
AB	A Barri RPN

AGH
Anywhere General Hospital
MEDICATION
ADMINISTRATION
RECORD

4476392
Desmarais, Pierre
144 King St.
Anywhere,
Ontario

Allergies   *Penicillin sulfonamides*

Diagnosis   *Diabetes, PVD, cellulitis*

Date

PRN and STAT Medication	10/6/05 Time Dose Route	Init	11/6/05 Time Dose Route	Init	12/6/05 Time Dose Route	Init	13/6/05 Time Dose Route	Init	14/6/05 Time Dose Route	Init
Tylenol #3 tabs 1-2 po Q4H PRN	1000 tt	RS	0345 tt	AB						
	1530 tt	RS	0800 tt	RS						
	2200 tt	RS	1300 t	RS						
lorazepam 0.5 mg sl QHS PRN	2200	AB								
Dulcolax 5 mg po or supp QHS PRN	2200 po	AB								

FIGURE 7-2 MAR for PRN and STAT medications.

Figures 7-1 and 7-2 would mean preparing containers of glyburide 5 mg, Cardizem SR 90 mg, Ancef 1 g, Pravachol 40 mg, Dulcolax 5 mg tablets, and Dulcolax 5 mg suppositories. Typically, the pharmacy sends a one-week supply of all medications. The package is sent to the unit, where it becomes the nurse's responsibility to calculate and administer the right dosage at the right time.

Having the patient's name on the label—which, of course, you will always check—gives a measure of safety to this system, but it requires more calculation by the nurse and hence creates an increased risk of dosage error.

Stock Supply

One of the oldest and simplest protocols is simply storing a supply of the commonly used medications on each unit. When the order is transferred to an MAR, the nurse calculates the dose, removes it from the container, and administers it.

Of all the systems, this one poses the greatest risk of error. A nurse could end up giving the wrong drug, the wrong dose, or both. To make things worse, medications are often stored in alphabetical order. That means if Lasix 20 mg and Losec 20 mg are side by side on the shelf, it's easy to pick up the wrong drug.

The stock supply system is rarely used as the only method for delivering medications. Not only does it introduce extra room for errors, it is expensive to keep large quantities of medication on each unit. It's probably for these reasons that some institutions use a stock supply system as a supplement to a unit dose or individual container protocol.

The rationale for a partial stock supply method is that it offers a way of ensuring the patient can start therapy immediately if it involves the common medications kept on the unit. A partial stock supply compensates for the fact that small institutions can't have a pharmacist on duty day and night. Another place where you might find a stock supply system is in emergency departments and clinics. They have a rapid turnover of patients, so they keep a dose or two of the usual medications to administer before a patient is discharged or transferred.

Because narcotics are frequently handled by a stock supply method, the unit's storage has to meet the standards of the Controlled Drugs and Substances Act. The narcotics cupboard is the place where restricted drugs are locked up. Each dose has to be documented as it is given, specifying the name of the patient, the drug, the dose, and the name of the nurse administering the medication. This record is in addition to the normal MAR. There are frequent checks (counts) to make sure the contents of the narcotics cupboard matches up with the documentation.

KEEP IT SAFE Stock supply systems have the fewest external checks on the medications you are administering. When you are taking medications from a stock supply, take extra care that you have the right drug, for the right patient, in the right dose, by the right route, and at the right time.

Computerized Systems

Everybody knows you can't do much these days unless you use a computer, and medication delivery is no exception. Along with payrolls and records, the computer can be used for a full or partial method of delivery. This may be a very simple approach, with the nurse sending requisitions to the pharmacy using the computer instead of paper. In more modern settings, the whole medication delivery protocol may be computerized.

You can handle the simple set-up, so let's take a look at the fully computerized ones. Usually, each patient has an electronic chart instead of a paper one, and the doctor enters any orders into this via computer. The system automatically notifies the pharmacy, the MAR is created and printed, and the pharmacist sets up the medication cart and sends it to the unit.

When you are ready to administer medications, you enter your password into the computer on the cart. You enter (or choose) the name of the patient and are presented with a list of his or her medications. You type in (or select) the medication you plan to give, and a drawer containing unit dose packages of that medication pops opens. You remove the package and administer the medication. You may sign for the drug on a paper MAR or by an entry into the computer.

Finally, some computerized systems use bar codes and hand-held scanners to identify the patient, the drug, and the nurse administering the drug.

Self Test

Answers to these questions are found at the end of the book.

1. Identify the components of a Medication Administration Record.

2. Which system provides a 24-hour supply of medication?

3. Which system usually provides a week's supply of medication?

4. Which system poses the greatest risk of error?

5. Which system may be used to supplement other systems?

means = extremes

Calculate the Dose

150 mg: A ml: 50 mg: 2 ml

(g/ml)

75 mg: A ml: 100 mg: 1 ml

75 mg IM QS PRN

Oral Medications

The student will:

- correctly calculate the dose of an oral solid using:
  - **Ratio and Proportion: Means = Extremes**
  - **Ratio and Proportion: Cross Multiplying Fractions**
  - **Formula**

- correctly calculate the dose of an oral liquid using:
  - **Ratio and Proportion: Means = Extremes**
  - **Ratio and Proportion: Cross Multiplying Fractions**
  - **Formula**

- **mix solutions correctly**

Dose: The amount of a drug that is to be given at one time, e.g., *50 mg of dimenhydrinate.*

Dosage: The amount of a drug plus the schedule on which it is to be given, e.g., *dimenhydrinate 50 mg Q4H PRN.*

Calculate the Dose

Once you have mastered the basic math and interpreted the doctor's order, you can go ahead and use the math to calculate the correct dose. Medications are usually ordered by weight. In the metric system, this is usually grams or milligrams.

Medications are manufactured so that a given weight of medication is in a given volume of the drug. This is the strength of the medication. For oral solids, the volume is 1 pill. Acetaminophen is manufactured in three strengths: 325 mg per pill, 500 mg per pill, or 650 mg per pill. When you receive an order for a given weight of medications, you must identify the strength of the medication and then calculate the volume or number of pills needed to administer that weight of drug.

Oral Solids

A large number of the medications administered by nurses are in the form of oral solids. Most of these are manufactured in the doses usually prescribed by doctors, so that only one pill has to be administered. Because of variations in patient age, size, and acuity, physicians may order more or less than the usual amount. This chapter will focus on the methods used to calculate the correct dose for each patient.

KEEP IT SAFE Because drugs are generally manufactured in the most common doses for adults, you should question any calculation that results in more than 3 tablets or less than $\frac{1}{2}$ tablet. To do this:

1. Check your math.
2. If the math is correct, check the doctor's order.
3. If the order has been transcribed correctly, find out if there are any special circumstances that would alter the usual dose. These circumstances might include unusual patient size, very severe illness or paediatric patients (see Chapter 16 for dosage calculation for children).
4. If there are no special circumstances, question the order with the physician.

Calculation Methods

There are three usual methods for calculating drug doses:

1. Ratio and Proportion: Means = Extremes
2. Ratio and Proportion: Cross Multiplication of Fractions
3. Use of a formula

Each of these methods is effective and accurate, so choose the one that works best for you.

KEEP IT SAFE No matter which method you choose for calculation, always begin by converting all of the elements to the same units. For example, if the order is for 1 g and the drug is available in 500 mg tablets, change the 1 g to 1 000 mg before beginning your calculations (see Chapter 1: Basic Math Review for the method for converting decimals).

EXAMPLE 8.1

The doctor's order reads: *Lasix (furosemide) 80 mg po OD*. The label on the stock (the bottle of Lasix) reads **Lasix 40 mg tablets**. We will use each of the above methods to calculate the appropriate dose of the drug.

FUROSEMIDE

Tablets

40 mg

100 Tablets

See full prescribing information for dosage and administration

Dispense in a tight, light-resistant container. Store at controlled room temperature 15-30°C.

Ratio and Proportion: Means = Extremes

(For review of the basic principles of Ratio and Proportion, see Unit 1, Chapter 2: Calculations Used in Determining Drug Doses. Recall that a ratio is a statement of the relationship of one quantity to another.)

When calculating oral solid doses, the relationship is between the number of mg (weight) of the drug and the number of tablets (volume). In the above example, the ratio of the stock—the *known ratio*—is 40 mg in one tablet, written as 40 mg : 1 tablet.

The ratio of the dose you have to give—the *unknown ratio*—is 80 mg to an unknown amount of tablets, written as 80 mg : A tablets.

A proportion is the relationship between two ratios. In this case, the unknown is equal to the known, written as $80:A = 40:1$

$$\downarrow\text{-means-}\downarrow$$
$$80:A = 40:1$$
$$\uparrow\text{-----extremes----}\uparrow$$

Multiply the means: $40 \times A$
Multiply the extremes: 1×80

Means equals extremes: $40A = 80$
Divide each side by 40: $A = 2$
Therefore the dose to be given is 2 pills.

Ratio and Proportion: Cross Multiplication of Fractions

When using this method, the ratio is stated in the form of a fraction.

The known ratio is 40 mg in 1 tablet, written as $\dfrac{40}{1}$.

The unknown ratio is 80 mg in A tablets, written as $\dfrac{80}{A}$.

Unknown equals known, so these fractions are equal: $\dfrac{80}{A} = \dfrac{40}{1}$

Cross multiply: $\dfrac{80}{A} \nwarrow \nearrow \dfrac{40}{1}$

$40A = 80$, or $A = 2$
Therefore the dose to be given is 2 pills.

Formula

Various formulae are available to calculate the quantity of a drug to give. One of the easiest is:

$$\frac{\text{Dose \textbf{D}esired (mg)}}{\text{Dose on \textbf{H}and (mg)}} \times \textbf{S}\text{tock (pills)} = \textbf{A}\text{mount (pills)} \ \text{ or } \ \frac{\textbf{D}}{\textbf{H}} \times \textbf{S} = \textbf{A}$$

Dose **D**esired is 80 mg.
Dose on **H**and is 40 mg.
Stock is 1 pill.

$$\frac{\textbf{D}}{\textbf{H}} \times 1 = \textbf{A} \qquad \frac{80}{40} \times 1 = \textbf{A}\text{mount}$$

Amount = 2 pills

EXAMPLE 8.2

The doctor's order reads: *Isoptin (verapamil) 120 mg po QHS.* The label on the stock (the bottle of Isoptin) reads **Isoptin 240 mg tablets.**

Ratio and Proportion: Means = Extremes

The known ratio is 240 mg : 1 pill.
The unknown ratio is 120 mg : A pills.
The proportion is 240:1 = 120:A.

$$\begin{array}{c} \downarrow\text{-means -}\downarrow \\ 240 \ : \ 1 \ = \ 120 \ : \ A \\ \uparrow\text{-------extremes--------}\uparrow \end{array}$$

Means: $1 \times 120 = 120$
Extremes: $240 \times A = 240A$

Means = Extremes: $120 = 240A$
Divide both by 240: $A = 0.5$, or $\frac{1}{2}$
You will give $\frac{1}{2}$ pill.

Ratio and Proportion: Cross Multiplication of Fractions

Known ratio is 240 mg in 1 tablet: $\dfrac{240}{1}$

Unknown ratio is 120 mg in A tablets: $\dfrac{120}{A}$

Unknown equals known, so these fractions are equal: $\dfrac{120}{A} = \dfrac{240}{1}$

Cross multiply: $\dfrac{120 \nwarrow \nearrow 240}{A \swarrow \searrow 1}$

$240A = 120$, or $A = \frac{1}{2}$
Therefore the dose to be given is $\frac{1}{2}$ tablet.

Formula

$$\frac{\text{Dose \textbf{D}esired (mg)}}{\text{Dose on \textbf{H}and (mg)}} \times \textbf{S}\text{tock (tablets)} = \textbf{A}\text{mount (tablets), or } \frac{\textbf{D}}{\textbf{H}} \times \textbf{S} = \textbf{A}$$

Dose **D**esired is 120 mg.
Dose on **H**and is 240 mg.
Stock is 1 pill.

$$\frac{(\mathbf{D})}{(\mathbf{H})} \times (\mathbf{S}) = \mathbf{A} \quad \frac{120 \text{ mg}}{240 \text{ mg}} \times 1 = \mathbf{A}$$

$$\mathbf{A} = {}^{1}/_{2} \text{ pill}$$

YOU TRY IT

(The answers to these questions are found at the end of the book.)

ORAL SOLIDS

1. The doctor's order reads: *ampicillin 750 mg po tonight, then 500 mg po QID for 10 days.* The label on the stock reads **ampicillin 250 mg capsules.**

   How many capsules will you give tonight? _____

   How many capsules per dose will you give tomorrow? _____

2. The doctor's order reads *digoxin 0.125 mg po OD.* The label on the stock reads **digoxin 0.25 mg tablets.**

   How many tablets will you give? _____

3. The doctor's order reads *Gravol (dimenhydrinate) 75 mg po Q4H PRN.* The label on the stock reads **Gravol 50 mg tablets.**

How many tablets will you give? _____

4. The doctor's order reads *trazodone 25 mg po QHS.* The label on the stock reads **trazodone 50 mg tablets.**

How many tablets will you give? _____

5. The doctor's order reads *Cardizem (diltiazem) 90 mg po BID.* The label on the stock reads **Cardizem 30 mg tablets.**

How many tablets will you give? _____

Oral Liquids

Oral liquids are used in a wide variety of situations. Patients who are unable to swallow pills may have liquids ordered or prepared for them; by the same token, pediatric medications are frequently liquid to make it easier for a baby to handle. Obviously, medications administered by nasogastric or gastrostomy tubes have to be in liquid form. There are also a few medications that are available in liquid form only.

KEEP IT SAFE It easy to become confused between the number of milligrams you are supposed to give and the number of milliliters you are supposed to give. The weight of the drug will be in milligrams. The volume of the drug will be in milliliters. Until you are comfortable with these calculations, write out the units (mg and ml) so you don't confuse them.

Calculating the amount of liquid medication to be given is much the same as calculating the number of pills needed. One of the traps awaiting the unwary is that you must be sure of the strength of the liquid. Most liquid medications are manufactured as a given number of milligrams in each milliliter of the liquid.

EXAMPLE 8.3

The doctor's order reads *Dilantin (phenytoin) 200 mg po TID*. The label on the stock reads **Dilantin Suspension 125 mg/5 ml**.

Ratio and Proportion: Means = Extremes

The known ratio is 125 mg : 5 ml
The unknown ratio is 200 mg : A ml
The proportion is 200 mg : A ml = 125 mg : 5 ml

$$\downarrow\text{-means-}\downarrow$$

$$200 \text{ mg} \; : \; A \text{ ml} \; = \; 125 \text{ mg} \; : \; 5 \text{ ml}$$

$$\uparrow\text{------------extremes-------------------}\uparrow$$

Means: $125 \times A = 125A$
Extremes: $200 \times 5 = 1000$
Means = Extremes: $125A = 1000$
Divide both by 125: A = 8 ml
You will give 8 ml of Dilantin

Ratio and Proportion: Cross Multiplication of Fractions

When using this method, the ratio is stated in the form of a fraction.
The known ratio is 125 mg in 5 ml:

$$\frac{125 \text{ (mg)}}{5 \text{ (ml)}}$$

The unknown ratio is 200 mg in A ml:

$$\frac{200 \text{ (mg)}}{A \text{ (ml)}}$$

Unknown equals known, so these fractions are equal: $\dfrac{200 \text{ (mg)}}{A \text{ (ml)}} = \dfrac{125 \text{ (mg)}}{5 \text{ (ml)}}$

Cross multiply: $\dfrac{200 \text{ mg}}{A \text{ ml}} \quad \dfrac{125 \text{ mg}}{5 \text{ ml}}$

$125A = 1{,}000$, or A = 8 ml
Therefore the dose to be given is 8 ml.

Formula

$$\frac{\text{Dose } \mathbf{D}\text{esired (mg)}}{\text{Dose on } \mathbf{H}\text{and (mg)}} \times \mathbf{S}\text{tock (ml)} = \mathbf{A}\text{mount (ml)}, \text{ or } \frac{\mathbf{D}}{\mathbf{H}} \times \mathbf{S} = \mathbf{A}$$

Dose **D**esired is 200 mg.
Dose on **H**and is 125 mg.
Stock is 5 ml.

$$\frac{D}{H} \times S = A \qquad \frac{200 \text{ mg}}{125 \text{ mg}} \times 5 \text{ (ml)} = A \text{ (ml)}$$

$$A = 8 \text{ ml}$$

EXAMPLE 8.4

The doctor's order reads *Lasix (furosemide)po 40 mg.* The stock is **Lasix elixir 10 mg/ml.**

Ratio and Proportion: Means = Extremes

The known ratio is 10 mg : 1 ml
The unknown ratio is 40 mg : A ml
The proportion is 40 mg : A ml = 10 mg : 1 ml

$$\downarrow\text{-means-}\downarrow$$

$$40 \text{ mg} \quad : \quad A \text{ ml} \quad = \quad 10 \text{ mg} \quad : \quad 1 \text{ ml}$$

$$\uparrow\text{----------extremes------------------}\uparrow$$

Means: $10 \times A = 10A$
Extremes: $40 \times 1 = 40$
Means = Extremes : $10A = 40$
Divide both by 10: $A = 4$ ml
You will give 4 ml of Lasix.

Ratio and Proportion: Cross Multiplication of Fractions

When using this method, the ratio is stated in the form of a fraction.

The known ratio is 10 mg in 1 ml : $\dfrac{10 \text{ (mg)}}{1 \text{ (ml)}}$

The unknown ratio is 40 mg in A ml: $\dfrac{40 \text{ (mg)}}{A \text{ (ml)}}$

Unknown equals known, so these fractions are equal: $\dfrac{40 \text{ (mg)}}{A \text{ (ml)}} = \dfrac{10 \text{ (mg)}}{1 \text{ (ml)}}$

Cross multiply: $\dfrac{40 \text{ mg}}{A \text{ ml}} \nwarrow \nearrow \dfrac{10 \text{ mg}}{1 \text{ ml}} \swarrow \searrow$

$10A = 40$, or $A = 4$ ml
Therefore the dose to be given is 4 ml.

Formula

$$\frac{\text{Dose } \textbf{D}\text{esired (mg)}}{\text{Dose on } \textbf{H}\text{and (mg)}} \times \textbf{S}\text{tock (ml)} = \textbf{A}\text{mount (ml) or } \frac{D}{H} \times S = A$$

Dose **D**esired is 40 mg.
Dose on **H**and is 10 mg.
Stock is 1 ml.

$$\frac{D}{H} \times S = A \qquad \frac{40 \text{ mg}}{10 \text{ mg}} \times 1 \text{ (ml)} = A \text{ (ml)}$$

$$A = 4 \text{ ml}$$

YOU TRY IT

(The answers to these questions are found at the end of the book.)

ORAL LIQUIDS

The doctor's order reads *Tylenol (acetaminophen) 160 mg po Q4H PRN.* Your well-stocked medication cupboard contains a wide variety of strengths of acetaminophen liquid. Calculate the amount of acetaminophen liquid you would give for each of the following strengths.

1. 80 mg/0.8 ml

2. 80 mg/2.5 ml

3. 80 mg/5 ml

4. 120 mg/5 ml

5. 160 mg/5 ml

CRITICAL THINKING

You are working in a walk-in clinic. Two-year-old Melissa has been brought in with an earache. After examining her, the doctor writes the above order. Her mother tells you that she has no Tylenol in the house and will have to buy some on the way home. She tells you that she is not sure which strength of Tylenol to buy.

What factors will you consider in making your recommendation?

What recommendation will you make?

Mixing Solutions

Some medications that are given as oral liquids are not very stable in the liquid form. These medications are usually manufactured in powdered form and have to be reconstituted when they are to be given.

MAKE A NOTE

Solute: the solid particles (drug)

Solvent: the liquid (usually water) in which the solute is dissolved

Solution: the combination of the solute and the solvent

The product information, which comes with the medication, will contain the information you need to mix the solution. It will tell you how much solvent to add to get a solution of a given strength. When you have mixed the solution and know the strength, go ahead and calculate the dose following the instructions above.

EXAMPLE 8.5

Doctor's order: *Apo-Cloxi (cloxacillin) 100 mg po QID*. The label on the stock bottle reads **Add 42 ml of water to make 60 ml of Apo-Cloxi 125 mg/5 ml.**

Ratio and Proportion: Means = Extremes

The known ratio is 125 mg : 5 ml.
The unknown ratio is 100 mg : A ml.
The proportion is 100 mg : A ml = 125 mg : 5 ml.

$$\downarrow\text{-means-}\downarrow$$

$$100 \text{ mg} : \text{A ml} = 125 \text{ mg} : 5 \text{ ml}$$

$$\uparrow\text{-----------extremes---------}\uparrow$$

Means: $125 \times A = 125A$
Extremes: $100 \times 5 = 500$

Means = Extremes : $125A = 500$
Divide both by 125: $A = 4$ ml
You will give 4 ml of Apo-Cloxi.

Ratio and Proportion: Cross Multiplication of Fractions

When using this method, the ratio is stated in the form of a fraction.

The known ratio is 125 mg in 5 ml: $\dfrac{125 \text{ (mg)}}{5 \text{ (ml)}}$

The unknown ratio is 100 mg in A ml: $\dfrac{100 \text{ (mg)}}{A \text{ (ml)}}$

Unknown equals known, so these fractions are equal: $\dfrac{100 \text{ (mg)}}{A \text{ (ml)}} = \dfrac{125 \text{ (mg)}}{5 \text{ (ml)}}$

Cross multiply: $\dfrac{100 \text{ mg}}{A \text{ ml}} \nwarrow \nearrow \dfrac{125 \text{ mg}}{5 \text{ ml}}$

$125A = 500$, or $A = 4$ ml
Therefore the dose to be given is 4 ml.

Formula

$$\frac{\text{Dose } \textbf{D}\text{esired (mg)}}{\text{Dose on } \textbf{H}\text{and (mg)}} \times \textbf{S}\text{tock (ml)} = \textbf{A}\text{mount (ml)} \quad \text{or} \quad \frac{\textbf{D}}{\textbf{H}} \times \textbf{S} = \textbf{A}$$

Dose **D**esired is 100 mg.
Dose on **H**and is 125 mg.
Stock is 5 ml.

$$\frac{\textbf{D}}{\textbf{H}} \times \textbf{S} = \textbf{A} \qquad \frac{100 \text{ mg}}{125 \text{ mg}} \times 5 \text{ (ml)} = \textbf{A} \text{ (ml)}$$

$$\textbf{A} = 4 \text{ ml}$$

Answers to these questions are found at the end of the book.

ORAL SOLIDS

In the space below each question, write the number of tablets or capsules you will give in order to administer the medication as written.

1. Doctor's order *Prevacid 30 mg po OD*. Stock **Prevacid 15 mg tablets.**

2. Doctor's order *Levodopa 150 mg op BID*. Stock **Levodopa 100 mg tablets.**

3. Doctor's order *Librium 30 mg po QHS*. Stock **Librium 10 mg capsules.**

4. Doctor's order *dimenhydrinate 25 mg po Q4H PRN*. Stock **dimenhydrinate 50 mg tablets.**

5. Doctor's order *Diabenase 125 mg po OD*. Stock **Diabenase 250 mg tablets.**

6. Doctor's order *Ceftin 1 gm po Q6H*. Stock **Ceftin 500 mg capsules.**

7. Doctor's order *digoxin 0.125 mg po OD*. Stock **digoxin 0.25 mg tablets.**

8. Doctor's order *digoxin 0.5 mg po OD*. Stock **digoxin 0.25 mg tablets.**

9. Doctor's order *digoxin 0.0625 mg*. Stock **digoxin 0.125 mg tablets.**

10. Doctor's order *Penicillin G 1 million units po Q6H*. Stock **Penicillin G 500,000 unit tablets.**

ORAL LIQUIDS

In the space below each question, write the number of ml you will give to comply with the order.

11. Doctor's order *Colace 100 mg po QHS PRN*. Stock **Colace syrup 20 mg/5 ml.**

12. Doctor's order *Zithromax 600 mg po Q6H*. Stock **Zithromax suspension 900 mg/22.5 ml.**

13. Doctor's order *Erythrocin 750 mg po Q6H*. Stock **Erythrocin suspension 250 mg/5 ml.**

14. Doctor's order *Apo-Cloxi 200 mg po Q6H*. Stock **Apo-Cloxi suspension 125 mg/5 ml.**

15. Doctor's order *Amoxil 600 mg po Q6H*. Stock **Amoxil suspension 250 mg/5 ml.**

16. Doctor's order *Gravol 25 mg po Q4H PRN*. Stock **Gravol liquid 15 mg/5 ml.**

17. Doctor's order *Benadryl 12.5 mg po Q4H PRN*. Stock **Benadryl Elixir 6.25 mg/5 ml.**

18. Doctor's order *dicyclomine 15 mg po QID*. Stock **dicyclomine syrup 10 mg/5 ml.**

19. Doctor's order *Kaon 40 mEq po BID*. Stock **Kaon liquid 20 mEq/15 ml.**

20. Doctor's order *Periactin 20 mg po QID*. Stock **Periactin Syrup 2 mg/5 ml.**

Parenteral Medications

The student will:

- correctly calculate the dose of a liquid parenteral medication using:
  - Ratio and Proportion: Means = Extremes
  - Ratio and Proportion: Cross Multiplying Fractions
  - Formula

- correctly calculate the amount of solvent to add to a small amount of liquid to facilitate accurate administration of a medication

- accurately identify the amount of solvent to add to a medication vial to reconstitute the medication

- correctly calculate the dose of a reconstituted medication using:
  - Ratio and Proportion: Means = Extremes
  - Ratio and Proportion: Cross Multiplying Fractions
  - Formula

Parenteral medication: medication that enters the body by some means other than the GI tract.

Ampoule/ampule: a sterile glass or plastic container that usually contains a single dose of a solution to be administered parenterally.

CPS (Compendium of Pharmaceuticals and Specialties): drug reference book published annually by the Canadian Pharmacists Association.

Vial: a glass container with a metal-enclosed rubber seal. It may contain a liquid or a powder and can contain one or more doses.

Diluent: liquid that is added to a powdered medication to make a solution suitable for injection.

Parenteral medications are administered by a route that bypasses the gastrointestinal tract. There are three main routes: injection, absorption through mucous membrane, and absorption through skin.

Medications may be administered by injection into subcutaneous tissue, muscle tissue, or into a vein, so these drugs must be in a liquid form. Some are manufactured in liquid form; but others come in a powdered form that has to be dissolved in liquid.

Liquid Preparations

Liquids for injection may be in ampoules or vials. An ampoule is a sterile glass or plastic container, usually containing a single dose of a solution (Figure 9-1). A vial is a glass container with a metal-enclosed rubber seal; it can contain enough medication for one or more doses (Figure 9-2). The strength of the medication will be stated on the

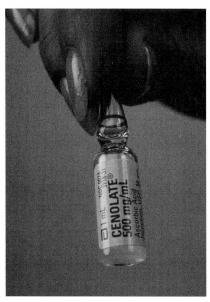

FIGURE 9-1 Ampoule. From Evans-Smith, P. (2005). *Taylor's clinical nursing skills: A nursing process approach* (p. 122). Philadelphia: Lippincott Williams & Wilkins.

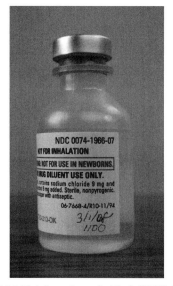

FIGURE 9-2 Vial. From Evans-Smith, P. (2005). *Taylor's clinical nursing skills: A nursing process approach* (p. 126). Philadelphia: Lippincott Williams & Wilkins.

ampoule or vial, e.g., **morphine sulphate 10 mg/ml.** The calculation of the dose is the same as for oral medications.

EXAMPLE 9.1

The doctor's order reads *Stemetil (prochlorperazine) 5 mg IM Q4H PRN.* The label on the ampoule reads **Stemetil 10 mg/2 ml.**

> **STEMETIL**
>
> **10 mg/2 ml**
>
> See full prescribing information for dosage and administration
>
> Dispense in a tight, light-resistant container. Store at controlled room temperature 15-30°C.

Ratio and Proportion: Means = Extremes

The known ratio is 10 mg : 2 ml
The unknown ratio is 5 mg : A ml
The proportion is 5 mg : A ml = 10 mg : 2 ml

↓-means-↓

5 mg : A ml = 10 mg : 2 ml

↑-------extremes----------↑

Means = $10 \times A = 10A$
Extremes = $5 \times 2 = 10$

Means = Extremes $10A = 10$
Divide both by 10
A = 1 ml
You will give 1 ml of Stemetil.

Ratio and Proportion: Cross Multiplication of Fractions

When using this method, the ratio is stated in the form of a fraction.
The known ratio is 10 mg in 2 ml

This is written $\dfrac{10\,(mg)}{2\,(ml)}$

The unknown ratio is 5 mg in A ml

This is written $\dfrac{5\,(mg)}{A\,(ml)}$

Unknown equals known, so these fractions are equal: $\dfrac{5\,(mg)}{A\,(ml)} = \dfrac{10\,(mg)}{2\,(ml)}$

Cross multiply: $\dfrac{5\,mg}{A\,ml} \nwarrow \nearrow \dfrac{10\,mg}{2\,ml}$

$10A = 10$, or A = 1 ml
Therefore the dose to be given is 1 ml.

Formula

$$\frac{\text{Dose \textbf{D}esired (mg)}}{\text{Dose on \textbf{H}and (mg)}} \times \textbf{S}\text{tock (ml)} = \textbf{A}\text{mount (ml) or } \frac{\textbf{D}}{\textbf{H}} \times \textbf{S} = \textbf{A}$$

Dose **D**esired is 5 mg
Dose on **H**and is 10 mg
Stock is 2 ml

$$\frac{\textbf{D}}{\textbf{H}} \times \textbf{S} = \textbf{A} \qquad \frac{5 \text{ mg}}{10 \text{ mg}} \times 2 \text{ (ml)} = \textbf{A} \text{ (ml)}$$

$$\textbf{A} = 1 \text{ ml}$$

YOU TRY IT

(The answers to these questions are found at the end of the book.)

LIQUID PREPARATIONS

1. The doctor's order reads *Demerol (meperidine) 75 mg IM Q3H PRN*. The label on the ampoule reads **Demerol 100 mg/ml**. How much Demerol will you give?

2. The doctor's order reads *Largactil (chlorpromazine) 150 mg IM TID*. The label reads **Largactil 50 mg/2 ml**. How much Largactil will you give?

LARGACTIL

See full prescribing information for dosage and administration

Dispense in a tight, light-resistant container. Store at controlled room temperature 15-30°C.

50 mg/2 ml

3. The doctor's order reads *Zantac (ranitidine) 50 mg IV BID*. The label reads **Zantac 25 mg/ml**. How much Zantac will you give?

4. The doctor's order reads *Valium (diazepam) 2.5 mg IV push Stat*. The label reads **Valium 5 mg/ml**. How much Valium will you give?

5. The doctor's order reads *Gravol (dimenhydrinate) 12.5 mg IM Q4H PRN*. The label reads **Gravol 50 mg/ml**. How much Gravol will you give?

Diluting Small-Dose Liquids

Sometimes the amount of liquid to be given by injection is very small. When a drug has a wide dosage range, the amount to be given at the lower end of the range may be difficult to measure. For example, morphine is usually packaged in ampoules of 10 mg/ml or 15 mg/ml. Some patients may have an order for *morphine 1 mg IV push*. Using the above calculations, the nurse would administer 0.1 ml of the drug.

The usual practice is to dilute 1 ml of the drug with 9 ml of normal saline or sterile water for injection. The concentration is then 1/10 of the original concentration. The strength is now 1 mg/ml, which can be easily measured.

To dilute small-dose liquids, the easiest method is to draw up 1 ml of the drug in a 10-ml syringe. You can then draw up 9 ml of sterile normal saline or sterile water into the same syringe. With a concentration of 1 mg/ml, you can use one of the usual calculation methods to determine the correct volume to administer.

KEEP IT SAFE Before diluting small-dose liquids, always check the package insert or the CPS (Compendium of Pharmaceuticals and Specialties) to ensure that there is no contraindication. There are some drugs that must not be diluted.

Reconstituting Powders

Many injectable medications are unstable in their liquid form, so they are packaged in powder form in glass vials. When you need to administer them, liquid is added to make a solution of a given strength.

The liquids usually added to powdered medication are sterile water for injection or sterile normal saline (0.9% saline) for injection.

KEEP IT SAFE Always read the label of the liquid you are using for reconstituting powdered medications and ensure that it states "for injection" or "injectable" on the label.

Some medications can't be diluted with sterile water or normal saline. In most cases these medications are packaged with the diluent. For example, *Solu-Cortef (hydrocortisone sodium succinate)* is diluted with a water and alcohol solution, which is in the same package as the powdered drug.

The amount and type of diluent for each powdered medication is usually identified in the package insert from the manufacturer. It will also tell you the strength of the reconstituted medication. If the package insert is missing, check it in the CPS.

Some medications may be diluted with different amounts of diluent, depending on the route and the final concentration desired. *Rocephin (ceftriaxone)* can be diluted with normal saline, sterile water, or 5% dextrose. These tables show the amounts of diluent and the resulting concentrations of the solutions.

ROCEPHIN
REGULAR VOLUME RECONSTITUTION TABLE (IM)

Vial Size	Volume to Be Added to Vial (ml)	Approximate Available Volume (ml)	Approximate Average Concentration (g/ml)
0.25 g	0.9	1	0.25
1.0 g	3.3	4	0.25
2.0 g	6.6	8	0.25

ROCEPHIN
LOW VOLUME RECONSTITUTION TABLE (IM)

Vial Size	Volume to Be Added to Vial (ml)	Approximate Available Volume (ml)	Approximate Average Concentration (g/ml)
0.25 g	not recommended for this vial size		
1.0 g	2.2	2.8	0.35
2.0 g	4.4	5.6	0.35

ROCEPHIN
RECONSTITUTION TABLE (IV)

Vial Size	Volume to Be Added to Vial (ml)	Approximate Available Volume (ml)	Approximate Average Concentration (g/ml)
0.25 g	2.4	2.5	0.1
1.0 g	9.6	10.1	0.1
2.0 g	19.2	20.5	0.1

CRITICAL THINKING

Sarah Kovacks is a 66-year-old woman who is 130 cm tall and weighs 46 kg. John Lee is a 48-year-old man who is 180 cm tall and weighs 80 kg. Each of them is to get 1 g of Rocephin IM.

Would you use the same amount of diluent for these two patients?

What factors would you consider in making this decision?

What further assessment should you carry out before making this decision?

What problems are the low volume reconstitution likely to cause for your patients?

What problems are the regular reconstitution likely to cause for your patients?

The technique for reconstituting a powdered drug in a vial is as follows:

- Wash your hands.
- Assemble your supplies, including the following:
  • the vial of drug
  • a container of the appropriate diluent
  • a syringe large enough to contain all of the diluent
  • an 18-gauge needle
  • alcohol wipes
- If there is a cap on the vial or the diluent, remove it. If there is no cap, wipe the surface with an alcohol wipe.
- Pierce the centre of the rubber stopper of the vial and remove an amount of air equal to the amount of liquid you will be adding.
- If the diluent is in a vial, inject the air into it. If the diluent is not in a vial, empty the syringe of the air.
- Withdraw the appropriate amount of diluent from the container.
- Inject the diluent into the medication vial.
- Remove the needle and rotate the vial until the powder is dissolved.
- Insert the needle into the vial and remove the appropriate amount of solution.
- If the vial is not going to be used immediately, or if it is a multidose vial, label the vial with the following information:
  • date
  • time
  • amount and type of diluent
  • strength of the resulting solution
  • your initials
- Wash your hands and discard any waste material.

The above technique is used for both single dose and multidose vials. When mixing a multidose vial, it is important that you write the data on the label, so when the vial is used later, its strength is accurately known.

The strength of a properly reconstituted vial of powdered medication will be part of the package information. This is used to calculate the amount of medication to give when you are not giving the entire vial in one dose.

MAKE A NOTE ✔

When you add a given amount of diluent to a vial containing powder, the amount of solution produced is usually greater than the amount of diluent you added. In the example below, 2.5 ml of sterile water is added to a vial of Ancef, producing 3 ml of solution. This is because the powder makes up part of the solution.

That's why you use the manufacturer's directions for mixing, rather than choosing an arbitrary amount.

EXAMPLE 9.2

The doctor's order reads *Ancef (cefazolin) 500 mg IV Q8H*. The label on the vial reads **Ancef 1 g**. You must reconstitute the Ancef and give the correct amount. The reconstitution directions read as follows:

Vial Size (mg)	Diluent	Volume to Be Added to Vial (ml)	Approximate Available Volume (ml)	Nominal Concentration (mg/ml)
1 000 mg	Sterile water for injection	2.5	3.0	334

Ratio and Proportion: Means = Extremes

The known ratio is 334 mg : 1 ml.
The unknown ratio is 500 mg : A ml.
The proportion is 500 mg : A ml = 334 mg : 1 ml.

$$\downarrow\text{-means-}\downarrow$$

$$500\ \text{mg} : \text{A ml} = 334\ \text{mg} : 1\ \text{ml}$$

$$\uparrow\text{------------extremes------------}\uparrow$$

Means = $334 \times A = 334A$
Extremes = $500 \times 1 = 500$

Means = Extremes : $334A = 500$
Divide both by 334
$A = 1.5$ ml
You will give 1.5 ml of the reconstituted Ancef.

Ratio and Proportion: Cross Multiplication of Fractions

When using this method, the ratio is stated in the form of a fraction.
The known ratio is 334 mg in 1 ml.

This is written $\dfrac{334\ (\text{mg})}{1\ (\text{ml})}$

The unknown ratio is 500 mg in A ml

This is written $\dfrac{500\ (\text{mg})}{1\ (\text{ml})}$

Unknown equals known, so these fractions are equal: $\dfrac{334\ (\text{mg})}{\text{A (ml)}} = \dfrac{500\ (\text{mg})}{1\ (\text{ml})}$

Cross multiply: $\dfrac{334\ (\text{mg})}{\text{A (ml)}} \nwarrow \nearrow \dfrac{500\ (\text{mg})}{1\ (\text{ml})}$

$500A = 334$, or $A = 1.5$ ml
The dose to be given is 1.5 ml.

Formula

$$\frac{\text{Dose \textbf{D}esired (mg)}}{\text{Dose on \textbf{H}and (mg)}} \times \textbf{S}\text{tock (ml)} = \textbf{A}\text{mount (ml)}\ \text{or}\ \frac{\textbf{D}}{\textbf{H}} \times \textbf{S} = \textbf{A}$$

Dose **D**esired is 500 mg.
Dose on **H**and is 334 mg.
Stock is 1 ml.

$$\frac{D}{H} \times S = A \qquad \frac{500 \text{ mg}}{334 \text{ mg}} \times 1 \text{ ml} = A \text{ ml}$$

$$A = 1.5 \text{ ml}$$

YOU TRY IT

(The answers to these questions are found at the end of the book.)

RECONSTITUTING POWDERS

1. The doctor's order reads *Tazidime (ceftazidime) 750 mg IV Q8H*. The label on the vial reads **Tazidime 2 g**. The reconstitution table reads as follows:

Vial Size (mg)	Diluent	Volume to Be Added to Vial (ml)	Approximate Available Volume (ml)	Nominal Concentration (mg/ml)
2 g	Sterile water for injection	10	11.2	180

How much of the solution will you give for each dose?

How many doses will this vial provide?

2. The doctor's order reads *cefotetan 600 mg IV Q12H*. The label on the vial reads **cefotetan 1 gm**. The label also states that the vial should be diluted with 10 ml of sterile water for injection yielding a concentration of 95 mg/ml. How much solution will you give for each dose?

3. The doctor's order reads *Pipracil (piperacillin) 1 g IM Q6H.* The label on the vial reads **Pipracil 2 g.** The reconstitution directions on the label read: add 4 ml sterile water for injection. Approximate concentration 0.4 g/ml. How much will you give?

4. The doctor's order reads *Mefoxin (cefoxitin) 1.5 g IV Q8H.* You have **Mefoxin 1 g** vials and **Mefoxin 2 g** vials available. The reconstitution table is as follows:

Vial Size	Diluent	Volume to Be Added to Vial (ml)	Approximate Available Volume (ml)	Nominal Concentration (mg/ml)
1 g	Sterile water for injection or 0.9% sodium chloride injection	10	10.5	95
2 g	Sterile water for injection or 0.9% sodium chloride injection	10	11.1	180

If you use two 1 g vials, how much solution will you draw up in total?

If you use the 2 g vial, how much solution will you draw up in total?

 CRITICAL THINKING

What factors will you take into consideration in deciding whether to use two 1 g vials or one 2 g vial?

Self Test

Answers to these questions are found at the end of the book.

LIQUID PREPARATIONS

In the space below the questions, write the number of ml you will give.

1. Doctor's order *Isoptin (verapamil) 7.5 mg slow IV push stat.* Stock **Verapamil 2.5 mg/2 ml.**

2. Doctor's order *Dilantin (phenytoin) 100 mg IM Q4H × 24 hours.* Stock **phenytoin injection 50 mg/ml.**

3. Doctor's order *thiamine 100 mg IM QAM.* **Stock thiamine 1 000 mg/10 ml.**

4. Doctor's order *Toradol (keterolac) 25 mg IM Q4H PRN*. Stock **Toradol 30 mg/ml.**

	See full prescribing information for dosage and administration
TORADOL	
30 mg/ml	Dispense in a tight, light-resistant container. Store at controlled room temperature 15-30°C.

5. Doctor's order *gentamycin 60 mg IV Q8H*. Stock **gentamycin 40 mg/ml.**

	See full prescribing information for dosage and administration
GENTAMYCIN	
40 mg/ml	Dispense in a tight, light-resistant container. Store at controlled room temperature 15-30°C.

6. Doctor's order *morphine 12 mg SC Q3H PRN.* Stock **morphine 15 mg/ml.**

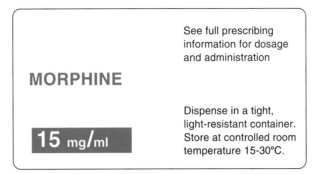

7. Doctor's order *Stemetil (prochlorperazine) 2.5 mg IM Q4H PRN.* Stock **Stemetil 10 mg/2 ml.**

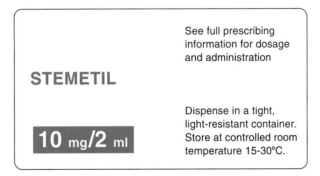

8. Doctor's order *Vitamin B₁₂ 2 mg IM each month*. Stock **Vitamin B₁₂ 100 mcg/ml.**

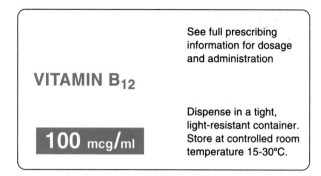

9. Doctor's order *Demerol (meperidine) 125 mg IM Q3H PRN*. Stock **Demerol 75 mg/ml.**

10. Doctor's order *Dilaudid (hydromorphone) 1 mg Q2H PRN*. Stock **hydromorphone 2 mg/ml.**

RECONSTITUTING POWDERS

In the space below the questions, write the number of ml you will give.

11. Doctor's order *Maxipime (cefepime) 0.5 g IM Q12H X 7 days*. Stock **Maxipime 1 g vial.** Add 2.4 ml sterile water for injection. Approximate concentration 280 mg/ml.

12. Doctor's order *Zinacef (cefuroxime) 1 g IV Q8H.* Stock **Zinacef 750 mg vials.** Add 8 ml sterile water for injection. Approximate concentration 90 mg/ml.

13. Doctor's order *Fortaz (ceftazidime) 1.5 g IV Q12H.* Stock **Fortaz 1 g vials.** Add 10 ml sterile water for injection. Approximate concentration 100 mg/ml.

14. Doctor's order *Ancef (cefazolin) 1 g IV Q8H.* Stock **Ancef 500 mg vials.** Add 2 ml sodium chloride for injection. Approximate concentration 225 mg/ml.

15. Doctor's order *Zovirax (acyclovir) 600 mg IV Q8H X 7 days.* Stock **Zovirax 1 g vial.** Add 20 ml sterile water for injection. Approximate concentration 50 mg/ml.

Administer the Medications

150 mg: A ml: 50 mg: 2 ml

(g/ml)

75 mg: A ml: 100 mg: 1 ml

Preparation of Oral Medications for Administration

The student will:

- **describe selected oral solids**

- **identify the types of oral solids that can be crushed or broken, and those that cannot**

- **describe the correct procedure for administering:**
  - **Oral solids**
  - **Crushed solids**
  - **Liquid medications**

Tablet: powdered medication and an inert substance that have been compressed into a small hard disc.

Capsule: medication that is inside a gelatine covering.

Enteric-coated tablet: tablets that have a protective coating that is resistant to stomach acids.

Extended-release tablet or capsule: tablet or capsule that has been formulated to release its contents slowly. These medications are active for a longer period of time than regular medications and so do not have to be taken as frequently.

The most common way of giving medications is by mouth. It offers several benefits. It is not invasive and does not usually cause pain to the patient. Very little in the way of specialized equipment is needed and most patients find it relatively easy to self-medicate. There are, however, some problems posed by oral administration. Some patients find it difficult to swallow oral solids and not all oral medications can be crushed in order to accommodate this. The patient must also have an intact and functioning gastrointestinal tract in order to absorb the oral medication. Many medications have adverse effects on the gastrointestinal tract. Patients who have gastrointestinal problems may not be able to tolerate these medications when they are given orally.

Types of Oral Solids

There are two major types of oral solids: tablets and capsules. Tablets are often referred to as pills.

Tablets are flat discs of compressed powder that contain the medication and a variety of inert materials that hold the tablet together. Some tablets are formulated to dissolve quickly, others to dissolve more slowly. Plain tablets usually have a slightly chalky or dusty surface and may be scored to facilitate breaking them into half-doses. Most plain tablets dissolve in the stomach, where they are absorbed through the mucosa into the vascular system.

There is also a variety of coated tablets. These have a smooth, shiny appearance. Some tablets have a light coating that makes them easier to swallow. Most coated tablets have a heavier, enteric coating. There are two major reasons for enteric coating. Some drugs such as NSAIDs (nonsteroidal anti-inflammatory drugs) are locally destructive to the mucosa of the stomach. They cause less damage if they dissolve in the duodenum. Other drugs are not well absorbed in the highly acid medium of the stomach. The pH of the duodenum and the jejunum is higher than that of the stomach, allowing more of the drug to be absorbed.

KEEP IT SAFE Tablets are manufactured in a wide variety of shapes and colours. Do not use only the shape and colour to identify the drug you are giving. The tablet of a specific drug manufactured by one company will look quite different from that manufactured by another company. Many hospitals and community agencies buy their drugs from whichever company offers them the best price at the time, so the pink tablet you give today may be blue or yellow tomorrow.

Capsules are small gelatine containers holding a single dose of powdered, granulated, or liquid medication. Capsules that contain powders or granules are usually made in two parts and can be taken apart and the powder or granules poured out if necessary. Capsules containing liquids are in one piece and cannot be taken apart. Half doses of capsules are not possible because of the difficulty of measuring the amount of powder accurately.

Caplets are tablets that have a light coating and are shaped to look like a capsule. Some patients find them easier to swallow than round tablets.

Administering Oral Solids

When you have calculated the correct dose of an oral medication, you should pour it into a paper or plastic medication cup before giving it to the patient. Do not touch it with your fingers. If it must be broken in half, use a scalpel or a pill cutter so that the division is even. Usually, all of the medications due at the same time can be placed in the same cup. Exceptions to this are medications that require a nursing assessment immediately before administration. For example, you should take the patient's blood pressure before you give antihypertensives. You should put these medications into a separate medication cup because you may withhold them as a result of the assessment. Take the medications to the patient's bedside, check the arm band, and hand the patient the medication cup and a cup of water. Stay with the patient until the medication has been swallowed.

MAKE A NOTE ✔

Some patients find it difficult to swallow tablets or capsules. To make it easier, put the tablet on top of a half-spoonful of applesauce or pudding. Tell the patient to swallow the tablet and the applesauce together without chewing. This procedure works best if done one tablet at a time.

KEEP IT SAFE **Always check the patient's allergies before administering any medication. This information should be assessed on admission and documented on the chart and on the MAR. If there is no documentation, ask the patient if he or she has any allergies before administering medications. Keep in mind that patients may be allergic to the inert portion of the medication or to the colouring agent. The CPS identifies some of the most common allergens found in medications in the purple pages.**

To Crush or Not to Crush

Some patients are completely unable to swallow oral solids; others have a feeding tube and can only take in liquids. In these cases, the usual practice is to crush the medications and dissolve them in a small amount of liquid. Capsules can be taken apart and the contents dissolved.

It is difficult to find concise, readily accessible information about whether or not an oral solid can be crushed or broken. There are some types of oral solids that definitely should *not* be crushed or broken. These include:

- Enteric-coated tablets: Crushing or breaking these destroys the coating and defeats the purpose of the coating. In addition, crushing these tablets results in hard, broken bits of coating that can injure the oral mucosa.
- Extended-release tablets or capsules: Crushing or breaking the tablets results in the release of the whole dose at one time, potentially causing an overdose. Some extended-release tablets are scored. These can be broken along the score line, but they may not be crushed, e.g., *Isoptin (verapamil) 240 mg tabs*. Most extended-release capsules should be swallowed whole, but there are some that can be opened and the granules emptied onto a spoonful of applesauce. These granules should be swallowed whole without chewing.

Any tablet that is scored can be broken along the score line. If these tablets are <u>not</u> extended release, they may also be crushed. Unscored tablets without enteric coating can usually be crushed, but the best practice is to check the individual drug.

There are several sources of information about crushing medications. The CPS is one of the best sources. The Clin-Info section (purple pages) contains a large Drug Administration and Food table that identifies a number of the medications that can and cannot be crushed. Nursing drug guides also frequently state whether or not a medication can be crushed or broken. If the information is not available from either of these sources, ask the pharmacist who filled the prescription to check the product information insert published by the manufacturer.

Administering Crushed Solids

There are a variety of methods for crushing tablets. The method you use will depend on the equipment available to you. If you have no equipment, place the tablet in the bowl of a spoon, place another spoon on top of it, and press down in a rocking motion until the tablet is crushed. If you have paper medication cups, put the tablet in one cup, put another on top, and rock the bowl of the spoon over the tablet until it breaks up. Both of these methods will work, but they are time-consuming and it is difficult to get very small pieces.

The commonest equipment for crushing tablets is the mortar and pestle (Figure 10-1). Place the tablet in the bowl of the mortar and crush it using the pestle. Some nurses use the pestle only to crush medication in a paper or plastic cup. There are also commercial tablet crushers available.

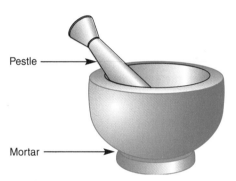

Pestle

Mortar

FIGURE 10-1 Mortar and pestle.

If you use a mortar and pestle or a commercial crusher, all of the medications for one patient can be crushed at the same time. It should then be washed before being used for another patient. It is not sufficient to simply wipe it out, as small amounts of medication can adhere to the equipment and get mixed into another patient's medications. Any equipment used in medication preparation should be washed after each use.

Two-part capsules are simply pulled apart and the contents emptied out. One-part gelatine capsules that contain liquids such as *docusate* or *chloral hydrate* should be placed in a small amount of warm water. The gelatine will dissolve and the medication will mix with the water.

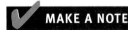
MAKE A NOTE

When it has been established that a patient will need to have medications crushed, you should contact the pharmacy and find out how many of the medications are available in liquid form. Liquids are easier and safer to administer than crushed solids. It is not necessary to get a doctor's order to use a liquid rather than a solid as long as the medication in question is not an extended-release preparation.

When administering crushed medications to a patient who is taking them by mouth, it is best to mix them with a small amount of a semisolid such as applesauce, pudding, jam, or honey. With patients capable of responding, let them choose what the medication will be mixed in. Mix the medication in the smallest amount of the semisolid possible.

Many medications taste very bitter and the patient may not be willing to take more than one mouthful. Have a glass of water or compatible fruit juice available as soon as the patient has taken the medication. Some fruit juices are not compatible with some medications. Grapefruit juice interacts with many medications and should be avoided.

Administering Oral Liquids

When preparing oral liquids, first determine whether or not the bottle of liquid should be shaken before pouring. As a general rule, cloudy liquids should be shaken, clear ones should not. Oral liquids are measured and administered in a graduated disposable plastic medication cup. The cup is held at eye level and the appropriate amount of liquid is poured into it. Because the cup is curved, the level of the medication also appears to be curved. The bottom of the curve (meniscus) should be at the level of the amount you wish to pour (Figure 10-2).

Some medications should be further diluted in water or compatible juice. Other liquid medications should be administered with a straw to avoid staining the teeth. Check your nursing drug guide for further information.

If at all possible, assist the patient to a sitting position before administering oral liquids. This will lessen the risk of the patient aspirating the medication.

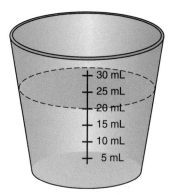

FIGURE 10-2 Medication cup.

Preparation of Injections for Administration

11

The student will:

- identify the appropriate volume of solution that may be given by subcutaneous injection

- identify the appropriate size of syringe and needle for subcutaneous injections

- identify the appropriate volume of solution that may be given by intramuscular injection

- identify the appropriate size of syringe and needle for intramuscular injections

- describe the appropriate technique for mixing two medications in the same syringe in the following circumstances:
  - medications from two ampoules
  - medications from one ampoule and one vial
  - medications from two vials

KEY TERMS

Subcutaneous injection (SC or Sub-q): injection that places the medications into the area below the dermis and above the muscle. For most patients, this area is approximately $\frac{1}{2}$ inch (1.25 cm) below the surface of the skin.

Sub-q set: a short length of tubing that has a half-inch needle on one end and a Luer-Lok or needleless connector on the other end. This is used to administer frequent doses of medications into subcutaneous tissue.

Intramuscular injection (IM): injection that places medication into the centre of a muscle.

Stat medications: medications that are to be given as soon as possible after being ordered by the physician.

Gauge: a number that identifies the size of the hole in a needle. Needles that have a higher gauge are thinner and have a smaller hole than needles that have a lower gauge. A 28-gauge needle is thinner than a 25-gauge needle. On the packaging of a needle, the gauge will usually be written 28G or 25G.

Overfill: most ampoules contain a slightly larger amount of drug than is identified on the label. This is to allow for the possibility of a small amount of spillage during preparation of the drug.

Luer-Lok: threaded connector on the end of a syringe or tubing. A needle that is twisted into a Luer-Lok connection will be held more firmly than one that is connected with a friction fit.

Ampule (ampoule): a single-use glass or plastic container for parenteral medications (Figure 11-1). The top is broken off to access the drug. If the entire amount of drug is not used, the remainder is discarded.

Vial: a glass or plastic container for parenteral medications that has a metal-enclosed plastic diaphragm on the top (Figure 11-2).

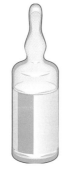

FIGURE 11-1 Ampoule.

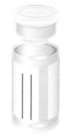

FIGURE 11-2 Vial.

There are a variety of reasons for giving medications by injection. Some medications are given subcutaneously because they cannot be absorbed through the GI mucosa. These include insulin and heparin, which are broken down by the digestive enzymes. Intramuscular injection is usually used for some stat medications, inoculations, postoperative analgesics and antiemetics, and medications for patients on whom it is not possible to start an IV. The administration of medication by injection has become less common in the past few years. Both subcutaneous and intramuscular injections are painful and some medications are traumatic to tissue. Many medications that were formerly given intramuscularly are now given by IV.

Syringes and Needles: Choosing the Appropriate Size

There are four routes used for the injection of medications: intradermal, subcutaneous, intramuscular, and intravenous. For preparation of intravenous medications, see Chapter 12.

Subcutaneous (SC or Sub-q) Injections

Subcutaneous injections place the medications into the area below the dermis and above the muscle. For most patients, this area is approximately $\frac{1}{2}$ inch (1.25 cm) below the surface of the skin. The subcutaneous tissue is fairly loose and is not well supplied with blood vessels. Absorption of medication from the subcutaneous tissue is slower than from muscle. If a large volume of medication is injected into the subcutaneous tissue, it may cause tissue damage before it can all be absorbed. For this reason, most authorities suggest that no more than 1 ml of medication should be injected at one time into subcutaneous tissue.

The choice of syringe for a subcutaneous injection depends on the amount of solution and the drug. If you are giving 1 ml of medication, it can be drawn up accurately in a 3-ml syringe. If you are giving less than 1 ml, it is difficult to get an accurate measurement in a 3-ml syringe because the graduations are not sufficiently exact. It is preferable to use a 1-ml tuberculin syringe that is marked in 0.01 ml increments (Figure 11-3).

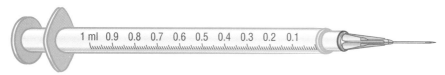

FIGURE 11-3 Tuberculin syringe.

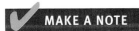
MAKE A NOTE

Canada uses the metric system for almost all measurements, but the United States does not. Some medical equipment that is imported from the United States continues to employ the Imperial system. One example of this is the length of needles used for parenteral injection. Single-use syringes that have attached needles are usually labelled with the volume of the syringe in millilitres, the diameter of the needle as the gauge (G), and the length of the needle in inches. It doesn't really make a lot of sense, but that is how it is. Thus a syringe that holds 3 ml of fluid and has a 25 gauge and a 5/8 inch needle will be packaged as "3ml25G5/8."

Recall that when measuring the gauge (diameter) of needles, the higher the number, the smaller the diameter.

For most patients, it is preferable to inject the medication $^1\!/_2$ inch or 1.25 cm below the skin. This can be accomplished by using a $^1\!/_2$ inch (1.25 cm) needle which is inserted at a 90° angle to the skin. It is best to use a small gauge needle—26 or 27 gauge—for most SC injections as these cause the least tissue trauma. Small gauge needles bend very easily. If the patient has very tough skin, or if the drug to be injected is thick or viscous, a $^1\!/_2$ inch, 27-gauge needle may be too fragile. In this case, a 5/8 inch, 25G needle should be used. If a 5/8 inch needle is used, it is inserted at a 45° angle to the skin so that the tip ends up $^1\!/_2$ inch (1.25 cm) below the skin.

Some patients require very frequent subcutaneous injections. Palliative patients may need narcotic analgesics every hour or oftener to maintain adequate pain control. Rather than puncture the patient repeatedly, you may decide to insert a sub-q set. This is a short length of tubing that has a $^1\!/_2$ inch needle on one end and a Luer-Lok or needleless connector on the other end. The tubing is primed with the medication and the needle is inserted into the subcutaneous tissue of the abdomen or upper arm. The needle is then taped in place and remains in the tissue for 3 to 5 days. When a dose of medication is required, it is drawn up in the usual manner and injected into the tubing. This system is more comfortable for the patient than repeated injections.

Sub-q sets may also be used with a continuous infusion pump to deliver small amounts of medication on a continuous basis. (See Chapter 13 for more information on continuous infusion pumps.)

Intradermal Injections

These injections place the medications into the dermis. They are used primarily for allergy and tuberculosis testing. When used for allergy testing, 0.05 − 0.1 ml of dilute allergen is introduced into the dermis. If the patient is allergic to the substance, a reddened wheal will form. Similarly in tuberculosis testing, 0.05 ml of a purified protein derivative of the tuberculosis bacillus is injected into the dermis. If the patient has antibodies to tuberculosis, a red, raised wheal will occur.

The amount of fluid used in these circumstances is very small, so a tuberculin syringe (see Figure 11-3) is used. This syringe is marked in 0.1 ml increments, making accurate measurement easier.

The needle only penetrates a very short distance below the skin, so a fine gauge, short needle such as 27G $^1\!/_2$-inch needle is most appropriate.

Intramuscular (IM) Injections

Intramuscular injections place medication into the centre of a muscle. The depth of an intramuscular injection varies with the size of the muscle and the amount of subcutaneous tissue that overlays the muscle. For most patients, a 1 $^1\!/_2$-inch needle is used to ensure that the tip is in the muscle, but the nurse should assess the patient and the injection site before choosing the needle. A 1-inch or 1 $^1\!/_4$-inch needle may be preferable for very thin patients, children or the deltoid muscle. If patients are very obese, a 2-inch or 3-inch needle may be necessary to reach the muscle. In most hospitals these can be obtained from the operating room where they are used by anaesthetists for spinal anaesthesia.

The amount of medication that can be injected in one dose also varies with the size of the patient and the site chosen. Most adults can tolerate up to 3 ml in one of the larger muscles such as the dorsogluteal, ventrogluteal, and vastus lateralus. No more than 2 ml should be given in the deltoid. Small adults and school age children may only be able to tolerate 2 ml, while younger children should only be given 1 ml IM.

The size of the syringe should be appropriate for the amount of fluid to be injected. Less than 1 ml may be drawn up in a tuberculin syringe. Tuberculin syringes are frequently packaged with 27G $\frac{1}{2}$-inch needles. This needle should be replaced with one suitable for IM injection. For amounts greater than 1 ml, a 3-ml syringe is usually used (Figure 11-4).

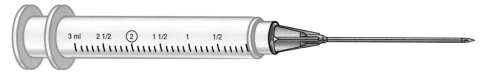

FIGURE 11-4 3-ml syringe.

It may be difficult to draw up a full 3 ml in a 3-ml syringe, in which case it is easier to use a 5-ml syringe.

Mixing Two Medications in the Same Syringe

There are times when the patient is to get two injections at the same time. If the drugs are compatible, two medications may be given at the same time in the same syringe. Two kinds of insulin may also be given together. The technique for drawing up two kinds of insulin in the same syringe will be found in Chapter 14.

There are also times when one container of medication may not be enough for the dose required.

KEEP IT SAFE When mixing two different drugs in the same syringe, it is important to check a drug compatibility chart to ensure that they can be mixed. Drug compatibility charts can be found in most nursing drug guides or posted on most hospital units. If one cannot be found, check with the pharmacist who dispensed the drugs.

Some frequently used combinations such as Demerol (meperidine) and Gravol (dimenhydrinate) are compatible for a short period of time only. If left in the syringe for too long, a precipitate will form. To avoid this, always administer these drugs immediately after mixing them.

When mixing two medications in the same syringe, calculate the volume of each drug using either the ratio and proportion or the formula method. (See Chapter 9 for the method for calculating the volume of drug to be given.) Add the two amounts to identify the total volume of medication that will be drawn into the syringe.

Medications from Two Ampoules

Read the labels of the ampoules and determine whether you will use all or part of each ampoule. If you require all of both ampoules, it doesn't matter which one you draw up first. Be aware that most ampoules contain a small amount of overfill, so when drawing up the first ampoule, take only the amount of drug required. When drawing up the second ampoule, pull the plunger of the syringe to the total amount previously calculated.

If you require all of one ampoule and part of another, the part ampoule should be drawn up first. This is because it may be more difficult to get exactly the right amount from a part ampoule than from a whole ampoule. When you have the correct amount in the syringe, you may then draw up the whole of the second ampoule.

The most difficult of the two-ampoule techniques is the situation where you need only a portion of each of two ampoules. It is best to draw up the smaller amount first. This is because smaller amounts are usually more difficult to measure than larger amounts. Draw up the smaller amount, then identify the total volume that should be in the syringe. Put the needle in the second ampoule and pull the plunger to the total volume.

Ampoules are single-use containers, so the same needle can be used for drawing up both drugs. Any unused portion of an ampoule should be discarded.

✔ MAKE A NOTE

When discarding partially-used ampoules of narcotics or other controlled drugs, make sure you have a witness and that appropriate documentation is carried out.

EXAMPLE 11.1

The doctor's order reads *meperidine 75 mg IM Q3H and prochlorperazine 5 mg IM Q3H PRN*. You have meperidine 100 mg/ml ampoules and prochlorperazine 10 mg/2 ml ampoules available.

Meperidine Calculation

Ratio and Proportion: Means = Extremes

Known ratio   100 mg : 1ml
Unknown ratio   75 mg : A ml
75 mg : A ml : 100 mg : 1 ml

$100A = 75$

$A = 0.75$ ml

Ratio and Proportion: Cross Multiplication of Fractions

Known ratio $\dfrac{100 \text{ mg}}{1 \text{ ml}}$

Unknown ratio $\dfrac{75 \text{ mg}}{A \text{ ml}}$

$\dfrac{75 \text{ mg}}{A \text{ ml}} \diagdown \diagup \dfrac{100 \text{ mg}}{1 \text{ ml}}$

$100A = 75$

$A = 0.75$ ml

Formula

$$\frac{\text{Dose \textbf{D}esired}}{\text{Dose on \textbf{H}and}} \times \textbf{S}\text{tock} = \textbf{A}\text{mount}$$

$$\frac{\textbf{D}}{\textbf{H}} \times \textbf{S} = \textbf{A} \qquad \bullet$$

D is 75 mg
H is 100 mg
S is 1 ml

$$\frac{75 \text{ mg}}{100 \text{ mg}} \times 1 \text{ ml} = \textbf{A} \text{ ml}$$

$$\textbf{A} = 0.75 \text{ ml}$$

You will draw up 0.75 ml of meperidine.

Prochlorperazine Calculation

Ratio and Proportion: Means = Extremes

Known ratio   10 mg : 2ml
Unknown ratio   5 mg : A ml
5 mg : A ml : 10 mg : 2 ml

10A = 10

A = 1 ml

Ratio and Proportion: Cross Multiplication of Fractions

Known ratio $\dfrac{10 \text{ mg}}{2 \text{ ml}}$

Unknown ratio $\dfrac{5 \text{ mg}}{A \text{ ml}}$

$$\frac{5 \text{ mg}}{A \text{ ml}} \diagup \diagup \frac{10 \text{ mg}}{2 \text{ ml}}$$

10A = 10

A = 1 ml

Formula

$$\frac{\text{Dose } \textbf{D}\text{esired}}{\text{Dose on } \textbf{H}\text{and}} \times \textbf{S}\text{tock} = \textbf{A}\text{mount}$$

$$\frac{\textbf{D}}{\textbf{H}} \times \textbf{S} = \textbf{A}$$

D is 5 mg
H is 10 mg
S is 2 ml

$$\frac{5 \text{ mg}}{10 \text{ mg}} \times 2 \text{ ml} = \textbf{A} \text{ ml}$$

$$\textbf{A} = 1 \text{ ml}$$

You will draw up 1 ml of prochlorperazine.
The total amount of drug in the syringe will be 1.75 ml.
Insert the needle into the meperidine and withdraw 0.75 ml.
Insert the needle into the prochlorperazine and withdraw until the amount in the syringe is 1.75 ml.

Medications from Two Vials

Read the labels on the vials and determine whether you will use all or part of each vial. The beginning steps of the procedure are the same whether you are using all or part of one or both vials.

- Reconstitute powdered medications according to the procedure in Chapter 9.
- Calculate the volume of drug to be withdrawn from each vial and add the two volumes to determine the total volume to be given.
- Inject air into each vial. In order to withdraw solution from a vial, it is necessary to first put air into it, so that you are not creating a vacuum when you withdraw the solution. The amount of air added should be the same as the amount of solution to be withdrawn. The vial should be in the upright position when adding the air. Make sure you do not touch the medication with the tip of the needle while injecting air. Air should be added to all of the vials before you start withdrawing solution from any of them. This decreases the chance of contaminating one vial with the solution in the other.

If you need all of the medication in both vials, remove the contents of one vial, and then the contents of the second vial. As with ampoules, if you are using all of both vials, it really doesn't matter which one you draw up first.

If you need all of one vial and part of another, draw up the part vial first, followed by the whole vial. Many vials are multiuse, so this protects the partly-used vial from contamination. The same needle can be used for both of the above procedures.

If only part of each vial is to be used, care must be taken to avoid contamination of one drug by the other. Draw up the smaller amount of drug into the syringe. Change needles, ensuring that there is no air in the syringe. Put the new needle into the second vial and draw up sufficient drug to equal the total volume that you previously calculated.

Medication from One Ampoule and One Vial

Read the labels on the ampoule and the vial and determine if you will use all or part of each. If necessary, reconstitute the powdered medication in the vial.

KEEP IT SAFE Do not use the liquid medication in an ampoule to reconstitute powdered medication in a vial. The resulting solution will be very concentrated and may cause tissue damage in the patient.

Inject the appropriate amount of air into the vial. If you are using all of both containers, withdraw the medication from the vial and then from the ampoule. If you take the medication from the ampoule first, the force required to pierce the rubber stopper of the vial may result in some of the solution in the needle being introduced into the vial.

The most common situation involves a single-use ampoule and a multiuse vial. Withdraw the appropriate amount from the vial, then withdraw medication from the ampoule. Draw up the amount necessary to equal the previously calculated total volume. It is not necessary to change the needle in this case. If not all of the ampoule is used, discard the remaining drug.

KEEP IT SAFE Medications for injection should always be checked for expiry date. It is also important to examine injectable liquids for discolouration, cloudiness or unusual precipitate. If you are not sure whether a colour or precipitate is normal, check with the pharmacist. Do not administer a medication you are unsure about.

EXAMPLE 11.2

The doctor's order reads *meperidine 100 mg IM Q3H PRN and dimenhydrinate 50 mg IM PRN.* You have meperidine 100 mg/ml ampoules and a multiuse vial of dimenhydrinate marked 250 mg/5ml.

  You will give the entire 1 ml ampoule of meperidine.

Dimenhydrinate Calculation

Ratio and Proportion: Means = Extremes

Known ratio   250 mg : 5ml
Unknown ratio   50 mg : A ml
50 mg : A ml : 250 mg : 5 ml

250A = 250

A = 1 ml

Ratio and Proportion: Cross Multiplication of Fractions

Known ratio $\dfrac{250 \text{ mg}}{5 \text{ ml}}$

Unknown ratio $\dfrac{50 \text{ mg}}{A \text{ ml}}$

$\dfrac{50 \text{ mg}}{A \text{ ml}} \quad \dfrac{250 \text{ mg}}{5 \text{ ml}}$

250A = 250

A = 1 ml

Formula

$$\frac{\text{Dose } \mathbf{D}\text{esired}}{\text{Dose on } \mathbf{H}\text{and}} \times \mathbf{S}\text{tock} = \mathbf{A}\text{mount}$$

$$\frac{\mathbf{D}}{\mathbf{H}} \times \mathbf{S} = \mathbf{A}$$

D is 50 mg
H is 250 mg
S is 5 ml

$$\frac{50 \text{ mg}}{250 \text{ mg}} \times 5 \text{ ml} = \mathbf{A} \text{ ml}$$

$$\mathbf{A} = 1 \text{ ml}$$

You will draw up 1 ml of dimenhydrinate.
The total amount of medication in the syringe will be 2 ml.

Inject 1 ml of air into the vial of dimenhydrinate.
Withdraw 1 ml of drug from the vial.
Draw up the entire vial (1 ml) of meperidine.
You will have 2 ml of medication in the syringe.

There are times when one container of medication may not be enough for the dose required. The same technique is used in drawing up the same medication from two containers as is used in drawing up two different medications.

Intravenous Therapy

The student will:

- identify the equipment used in administering intravenous (IV) solutions
- calculate the flow and drip rates for gravity IVs
- calculate the flow rate for IV pumps

Hydrostatic pressure: in the vascular system, the pressure exerted by the blood against the walls of the blood vessels.

Osmotic pressure: in the vascular system, the pressure that causes the movement of a solvent (water) from an area of low concentration of solute (particles such as plasma proteins and glucose) to an area of high concentration of solute.

Isotonic: a solution that will exert an osmotic pressure similar to that of blood plasma.

Hypotonic: a solution that will exert an osmotic pressure lower than that of blood plasma.

Hypertonic: a solution that will exert an osmotic pressure higher than that of blood plasma.

Flow rate: the number of millilitres of fluid administered over one hour (ml/hr).

Drip rate: the number of drops administered per minute (gtts/min).

Drip factor: the number of drops of IV solution per millilitre of fluid (gtts/ml).

Infusion time: the time required to infuse a specific volume of fluid.

Vascular access device: a catheter that is inserted into a vein or artery and can be used to instil fluids into the body or remove blood from the body.

Angiocatheter: short, flexible vascular access device that is inserted into a peripheral vein. It is usually 2.5 cm to 10 cm long.

Equipment Used in IV Therapy

Intravenous infusion to administer fluids, electrolytes, nutrients, and medications to the patient is a common practice in hospital settings and is becoming more so in community and long-term care settings. These elements can be administered into a peripheral vein or into the right vena cava through a central line. IV fluid moves into a patient's vein because the hydrostatic pressure is higher in the intravenous than it is in the vein. This pressure may come from gravity or from a pump. When gravity is used, hanging the bag of IV fluid higher than the patient's heart provides the appropriate pressure. When a pump is used, the pressure is provided by the machine. To provide IV therapy, you need vascular access devices, IV fluid, and IV tubing, which are discussed in the following sections.

Vascular Access Devices

An IV is established through a vascular access device that is inserted into one of the patient's blood vessels. Peripheral IV's are established when a short (2.5–10 cm) angiocatheter (angiocath) is inserted into a vein. It is preferable to use a vein in the arm or hand, but foot and scalp veins may be used in special circumstances.

Peripherally inserted central catheters (PICC) are much longer catheters that are inserted into a peripheral vein and threaded through the vascular system to the right vena cava.

Centrally inserted catheters are tunnelled through the subcutaneous tissue of the chest, inserted into a major vein, and directed into the right vena cava.

IVs may run continuously or intermittently. If they are run intermittently, the outer end of the vascular access device can be closed off or locked and the tubing attached as necessary. The portion of the vascular access device that is in the vein may stimulate the clotting mechanism, so locked access devices are usually flushed with normal saline or heparin on a regular basis to prevent clot formation.

IV Fluid

Most IV fluid is packaged in plastic bags (Figure 12-1). Most bags have two ports or access points. The primary port can be pierced with the spike on the end of the IV tubing. There is also an injection port, through which electrolytes and medications may be added. A few solutions are incompatible with plastic, and these will be packaged in glass bottles that are accessed through a rubber diaphragm similar to that on the top of a medication vial.

IV bags come in a variety of sizes, ranging from 50 ml to 1 000 ml. They are usually marked with a graduated scale along one side to make it easy to see how much fluid is remaining in the bag at any time. This information can then be used to calculate how much fluid the patient has received.

Bags are also marked with an expiry date that should be checked before hanging a new bag of IV fluid.

The bag is also labelled with the name and the contents of the solution. Most solutions contain sodium chloride, dextrose (a sugar), and/or electrolytes in a variety of strengths. There are several abbreviations used to identify the contents. NS stands for normal saline. This is 0.9% sodium chloride or 0.9 g of sodium chloride per 100 ml of fluid. Variations in the amount of sodium chloride are usually expressed as a fraction of "normal," e.g., 0.45% saline may be labelled 1/2NS.

The amount of dextrose in a solution is usually written as D5W. This means that the solution is 5% dextrose and water (5 grams of dextrose per 100 ml of water). D10W indicates 10% dextrose and water, while D5NS indicates 5% dextrose in normal saline.

Various solutions contain sodium chloride and electrolytes. Many of these are known by their proprietary names such as Ringer's Lactate and Normosol. Read the labels carefully, because some of the solutions are manufactured both with and without dextrose.

MAKE A NOTE ✔

In some settings, there is a convention in the naming of IV fluids that can be puzzling to the new practitioner. You may find that you get an order for "2/3 and 1/3" (two-thirds and one-third). You will not, however, find a bag of fluid with this label on it. The solution that has been ordered is actually 3.3% dextrose and 0.3% sodium chloride.

The nickname came about because at one time, the most common IV solution was 5% dextrose in normal saline. This solution is hypertonic and pulls water into the vascular system. It was determined that 2/3 of the customary amount of dextrose (or 3.3%) and 1/3 (or 0.3%) of the customary amount of normal saline would yield an isotonic solution. It is now a frequently ordered solution in many settings.

"Everyone" knows what 2/3 and 1/3 is, so the new practitioner must memorize the information since it is not actually written down anywhere.

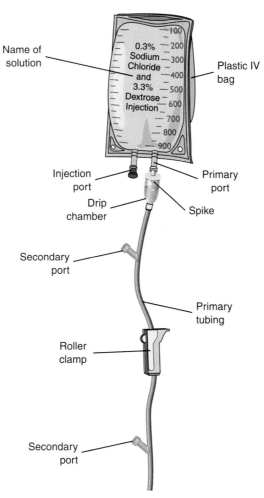

FIGURE 12-1 Intravenous equipment.

IV Tubing

The tubing that runs from the large bag directly to the patient is called the primary tubing. At the top of the IV tubing is the drip chamber. The spike at the top of the drip chamber is inserted into the bag through the primary port, so the IV fluid drips through the spike into the drip chamber. There are two sizes of drip chamber, macro

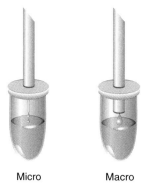

Micro   Macro

FIGURE 12-2 Drip chambers.

and micro (Figure 12-2). The macro drip delivers a larger drop than the micro. They can be differentiated by looking at the size of the opening at the top. The micro drip always delivers 60 drops per millilitre of fluid, but each manufacturer uses a slightly different diameter for the opening of the macro drip. As a result, each manufacturer's tubing delivers a drop of a slightly different size. These range from 10 drops/ml to 15 drops/ml. This becomes important when calculating the rate or number of drops per minute (gtts/min) at which the IV will run. The drip chamber should be kept about half full of IV fluid at all times.

The tubing extends from the drip chamber to the patient's vascular access device. The rate of flow of a gravity IV is controlled by a roller clamp. When the IV is on a pump, the pump controls the rate of flow. At one or more points along the primary tubing, there are secondary ports. These are used to establish a secondary or piggyback line or for the direct injection of medications.

KEEP IT SAFE IV therapy provides an open passageway from the outside to a patient's vascular system, so it increases the risk of infection. Strict surgical asepsis should be used when starting the IV, and whenever the solution and the tubing are changed. If a container of IV solution hangs for more than 24 hours, it should be changed whether it is empty or not. IV tubing should be changed according to agency policy, usually every 72 hours. It is important to assess the patient with an IV frequently for signs of potential infection. This should be part of the continuous assessment of these patients for all of the complications of IV therapy.

Flow Rates and Drip Rates

Calculation of Flow Rates and Drip Rates for Macro Tubing

Most IV orders direct you to give a patient a given amount of a specific solution over a given amount of time. In order to administer this correctly, you must be able to calculate the flow and drip rates.

Macro tubing is usually used for IVs when the amount of fluid to be given is more than 50–75 ml/hour, while micro tubing is used when the flow rate is less than 50–75 ml/hr. Either may be used when the flow rate is between 50 and 75 ml/hr.

EXAMPLE 12.1

The doctor's order reads *NS 1 000 ml IV Q8H.*

Flow rate is the number of millilitres of fluid administered over one hour (ml/hr). To calculate this, divide the amount of fluid by the number of hours over which it is to be administered.

$$\frac{\text{Amount of fluid (ml)}}{\text{Time in hours}} = \text{Flow rate (ml/hr)}$$

Drip rate is the number of drops administered per minute (gtts/min). In order to calculate the drip rate, you must know how many drops there are in 1 ml of fluid. This number is known as the *drip factor.* The drip factor varies from manufacturer to manufacturer, but is usually 10, 12, or 15 for most common tubing. The drip factor will be identified on the package of tubing. It is also necessary to convert the time from hours to minutes. To do this, multiply the number of hours by 60 minutes.

There are two methods for calculating drip rate. Both methods will use the above doctor's order and a drip factor of 15.

Two-Step Method

Step 1: Calculate the flow rate:

$$\frac{\text{Amount of fluid (ml)}}{\text{Time in hours (hrs)}} = \text{Flow rate (ml/hr)}$$

$$\frac{1\ 000\ \text{ml}}{8\ \text{hr}} = 125\ \text{ml/hr}$$

Step 2: Calculate the drip rate:

$$\frac{\text{Flow rate (ml/hour)}}{60\ \text{(minutes)}} \times \text{Drip factor (gtts/ml)} = \text{Drip rate (gtts/min)}$$

$$\frac{125\ \text{ml/hr}}{60} \times 15 = 31.25\ \text{gtts/min}$$

The IV will run at 31 gtts/min.

One-Step Method

Calculate the drip rate:

$$\frac{\text{Amount of fluid} \times \text{Drip factor}}{\text{Time in hours} \times 60\ \text{minutes}} = \text{Drip rate}$$

$$\frac{1\ 000\ \text{ml} \times 15\ \text{gtts/ml}}{8\ \text{hrs} \times 60\ \text{minutes}} = 31.25\ \text{gtts/min}$$

EXAMPLE 12.2

The doctor's order reads *2 000 ml D5W Q24H.* The drip factor for the tubing is 12 gtts/ml. Calculate the drip rate for this IV.

Two-Step Method

Step 1:

$$\frac{\text{Amount of fluid (ml)}}{\text{Time in hours (hrs)}} = \text{Flow rate (ml/hr)}$$

$$\frac{2\ 000\ \text{ml}}{24\ \text{hrs}} = 83.3\ \text{ml/hr}$$

Step 2:

$$\frac{\text{Flow rate (ml/hour)}}{60\ \text{(minutes)}} \times \text{Drip factor (gtts/ml)} = \text{Drip rate (gtts/min)}$$

$$\frac{83.3 \times 12}{60} = 16.6\ \text{gtts/min}$$

One-Step Method

$$\frac{\text{Amount of fluid} \times \text{Drip factor}}{\text{Time in hours} \times 60\ \text{minutes}} = \text{Drip rate}$$

$$\frac{2\ 000 \times 12}{24 \times 60} = 16.6\ \text{gtts/min}$$

Some physicians write IV orders using the flow rate rather than identifying a given amount of fluid over a given amount of time, e.g., *IV D5W @ 75 ml/hr. (Drip factor is 15.)* When this happens, the second step of the two-step method is used to calculate the drip rate.

$$\frac{\text{Flow rate (ml/hour)}}{60\ \text{(minutes)}} \times \text{Drip factor (gtts/ml)} = \text{Drip rate (gtts/min)}$$

$$\frac{75\ \text{(ml/hour)}}{60\ \text{(min)}} \times 15\ \text{(gtts/ml)} = 18.75\ \text{gtts/min}$$

When an IV is being used primarily to maintain access to a vein for medication administration, the order may be written "to keep the vein open" of TKVO or TKO. This means that the rate is set just fast enough to keep the IV flowing or patent. Generally this is considered to be approximately 30 ml/hr.

YOU TRY IT

(The answers to these questions are found at the end of the book.)

1. Doctor's order reads *D5W 1 200 ml IV Q8H*. Drip factor is 15. Calculate the drip rate.

2. Doctor's order reads *IV Ringer's Lactate 500 ml Q12H*. Drip factor is 10. Calculate the drip rate.

3. Doctor's order reads *IV 2/3 & 1/3 200 ml/hr for 12 hours, then 100 ml hr for 24 hours*. Drip factor is 12. Calculate both drip rates.

4. Doctor's order reads *IV NS 3 000 per day*. Drip factor is 15. Calculate the drip rate.

✔ MAKE A NOTE

Physicians sometimes write IV orders as a given amount of fluid per shift, e.g., IV 2/3 & 1/3 1 000 ml/shift. It used to be understood that a shift was the 8-hour period usually worked by the nursing staff. In recent years, many hospital units have changed to 12-hour shifts. Be sure to check agency policy regarding how many hours constitute a "shift" for the purposes of IV orders.

Calculation of Flow Rates and Drip Rates for Micro Tubing

Micro tubing is usually used when the flow rate is less than 50–75 ml/hour. It is also used in some secondary systems when administering IV medications.

When calculating the drip rate for micro tubing, it is best to use the two-step method. The calculation of flow rate is the same for micro tubing as it is for macro tubing.

$$\frac{\text{Amount of fluid (ml)}}{\text{Time in hours}} = \text{Flow rate (ml/hr)}$$

The calculation of the drip rate is simplified because the drip factor (60) and the minutes (60) cancel each other out.

$$\frac{\text{Flow rate (ml/hour)}}{60 \text{ (minutes)}} \times \text{Drip factor (gtts/ml)} = \text{Drip rate (gtts/min)}$$

Doctor's order reads *IV D5W 500 ml Q8H.*

Step 1:

$$\frac{\text{Amount of fluid (ml)}}{\text{Time in hours}} = \text{Flow rate (ml/hr)}$$

$$\frac{500 \text{ ml}}{8 \text{ hrs}} = 62.5 \text{ ml/hr}$$

Step 2:

$$\frac{\text{Flow rate (ml/hour)}}{60 \text{ (minutes)}} \times \text{Drip factor (gtts/ml)} = \text{Drip rate (gtts/min)}$$

$$\frac{62.5 \text{ (ml/hr)} \times \cancel{60} \text{ (gtts/ml)}}{\cancel{60} \text{ (minutes)}} = 62.5 \text{ gtts/min}$$

YOU TRY IT

(The answers to these questions are found at the end of the book.)

Each of these questions uses micro tubing.

1. Doctor's order reads *IV NS 300 ml/shift* (8-hour shift). Calculate the drip rate.

2. Doctor's order reads *IV D5W 400 ml Q8H*. Calculate the drip rate.

3. Doctor's order reads *IV Normosol M 1 litre Q24H*. Calculate the drip rate.

4. Doctor's order reads *IV 5% dextrose in normal saline 30 ml/hr*. Calculate the drip rate.

5. Doctor's order reads *IV D5W 400 ml Q12H*. Calculate the drip rate.

Calculation of Flow Rate for IV Pumps

It is not necessary to calculate a drip rate when using an IV pump. Most pumps simply require that you enter the flow rate and the pump takes care of it from there. The method for calculating flow rate for a pump is exactly the same as calculating the flow rate for a gravity IV.

Answers to these questions are found at the end of the book.

Calculate the drip rate for the following gravity IVs.

1. Doctor's order reads *IV NS 3 000 ml per day*. Drip factor is 10.

2. Doctor's order reads *IV 1 000 ml over the next 6 hours*. Drip factor is 15.

3. Doctor's order reads *IV D5W 1 000 ml per shift*. The shift is 8 hours. Drip factor is 15.

4. Doctor's order reads *IV Ringer's Lactate 60 ml per hour*. Drip factor is 12.

5. Doctor's order reads *IV 2/3 + 1/3 1 500 ml/ shift.* The shift is 12 hours. Drip factor is 12.

Calculate the drip rate for the following gravity IVs with microdrip tubing.

6. Doctor's order reads *IV 2/3 + 1/3 500 ml Q8H.*

7. Doctor's order reads *IV D5W 2 000 ml Q24H.*

8. Doctor's order reads *IV D5W 600 ml Q8H.*

9. Doctor's order reads *IV NS 40 ml/hr.*

10. Doctor's order reads *IV Ringer's Lactate 50 ml/hr.*

Calculate the flow rate for the following IV orders which are to be administered using an IV pump.

11. Doctor's order reads *IV NS 1 000 ml Q6H.*

12. Doctor's order reads *IV Ringer's Lactate 1 000 ml Q8H.*

13. Doctor's order reads *IV Normosol M 1 000 ml Q12H.*

14. Doctor's order reads *IV D5W 1 500 ml Q8H.*

15. Doctor's order reads *IV NS 500 ml Q12H.*

The student will:

- identify the equipment used in administering IV medications
- calculate the flow and drip rates for medications given by IV minibag
- calculate the flow and drip rates for medications given by IV soluset
- calculate dose/hour, dose/minute, and dose/kg/minute for medication given by continuous IV infusion
- describe portable continuous infusion pumps

IV Push: small quantity of intravenous medication that is injected directly into a vein.

Piggyback: secondary IV line that is attached to the primary line of an IV infusion set. It is generally used for medication administration.

Minibag: small (50–100 ml) bag of IV fluid used to further dilute IV medications.

Transfer needle/reconstitution device: a tool that enables the nurse to reconstitute a powdered medication and add it to a minibag at the same time. May also be used to add a liquid medication that is in a vial to a minibag.

Soluset: graduated cylinder that is attached to an IV bag and provides more precise control of volume and drip rate than the usual tubing.

Bolus: a dose of intravenous medication that is administered all at once.

The IV route is becoming an increasingly common method of medication administration. Medications administered by this route are absorbed very quickly and consistently.

There are a number of different ways medications may be administered intravenously. They may be administered intermittently or continuously. Intermittent administration can be carried out in several different ways.

Intermittent IV Medications

IV Push

Medications given IV push are injected directly into a vein, saline lock, or secondary port. Liquid medications are injected undiluted, while powdered medications are reconstituted according to the package insert. See Chapter 9 for the method for reconstituting powdered medications. Medications injected IV push are not usually diluted in a larger volume of fluid.

Minibag Used With Gravity IV

A minibag is a small IV bag that holds 50 to 100 ml of IV fluid. The medication to be administered is prepared and drawn up in a syringe and then injected into the minibag. Label the minibag with the name and dose of the medication, the time and date it was mixed, and your initials or signature. The minibag is attached to the primary tubing by a short piece of tubing that connects into a secondary port (Figure 13-1). This tubing is

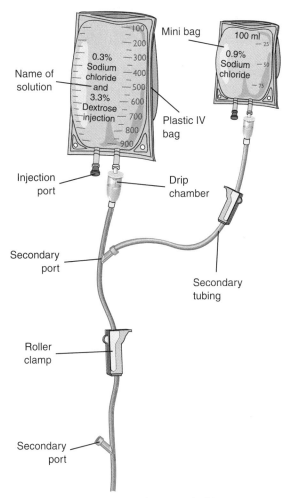

FIGURE 13-1 Minibag IV and tubing.

usually referred to as *secondary tubing*, or a *secondary line*. The minibag and tubing may also be called a *piggyback*.

The secondary line should be flushed with fluid from the primary bag. The first time the tubing is used, clamp the secondary tubing, push the spike into the minibag, and connect the other end of the secondary tubing to the highest secondary port on the primary tubing. Lower the minibag below the level of the primary bag and open the clamp on the secondary tubing. Fluid from the primary bag will flow into the tubing. When it half fills the drip chamber, clamp the tubing.

If the tubing has been in use and still contains some of the drug from the last medication, follow the same procedure, but allow the fluid to go right up into the empty bag. Clamp the tubing and then change bags. In this way, potentially incompatible medications will not come into contact with each other.

Before beginning to administer the medication, calculate the drip rate that will allow you to administer the contents of the minibag in the appropriate amount of time.

To administer the medication, lower the primary bag so that it is below the level of the minibag. When the minibag is higher than the primary, the minibag will run first. Open the clamp on the secondary tubing completely. Regulate the rate of flow using the roller clamp on the primary tubing. When the minibag is empty, the primary bag will resume dripping at the same rate that the minibag was running.

✔ MAKE A NOTE

Powdered medications that are in a vial can be reconstituted and added to a minibag at the same time using a transfer needle or reconstitution device. A transfer needle is a double-ended needle that has a plastic covering. The covering is designed to fit snugly over the vial at one end and the injection port of the minibag at the other end (Figure 13-2A). To reconstitute the medication, connect the transfer needle to the vial, and then to the minibag. Hold the connected pieces so that the minibag is up (Figure 13-2B). Squeeze the minibag until the vial is about half full of IV fluid. Rotate the bag and vial gently until the medication is mixed. Turn the connected pieces upside down so that the vial is up (Figure 13-2C). Squeeze and release the bag gently so that negative pressure forces air up into the vial and the reconstituted drug drains into the minibag. Label the bag appropriately and proceed as above.

Note: A transfer needle can only be used if all of the contents of the vial are to be added to the minibag. It cannot be used for partial or divided doses.

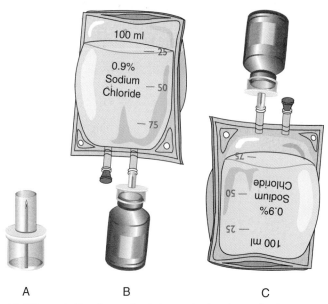

FIGURE 13-2 A, Transfer needle. B, Reconstituting the medication. C, Medication drains into minibag.

The decisions about what size of minibag and what kind of solution to use, and the rate at which an IV medication will run, require critical thinking and nursing judgment.

When deciding on the size of the minibag, consult the package insert and/or your nursing drug guide. These will give some information about what solution and size of minibag should be used. The information with some drugs is very specific and must be followed, but most drugs come with the direction "may dilute in 50–100 ml of usual IV fluids." This means that you must base your decision on your assessment of the individual patient and your knowledge of the drug. The factors that must be considered include the age, size, medical diagnosis, and hydration status of the patient, the condition of his or her veins, the number of IV medications he or she is getting, and the effect that the medication has on the veins.

The decision about the rate at which the medication will run also depends on your patient assessment and your knowledge of the drug. As well as the factors you considered when deciding the volume of the minibag, you also need to consider the rate at which the primary IV is running and the reason for that rate. For example, patients who need large volumes of fluid quickly should have a rapid rate of IV medication infusion. Patients who are at risk of fluid volume excess and who have a slow rate of IV infusion should receive their IV medications slowly as well.

CRITICAL THINKING

50-ml bags are usually preferable for small, elderly patients; those with medical diagnoses such as renal failure or congestive heart failure; those who are already overhydrated, and those with small veins. 100-ml bags are better for patients who are receiving drugs that tend to cause inflammation of the veins and those who are not well hydrated.

These are a few of the situations in which you would choose one size of bag rather than another. What other clinical situations would impact on the size of minibag you would choose?

Calculation of Drip Rate for Minibag Administration of IV Medications

The formula for calculation of drip rate for IV meds is similar to that for calculation of the primary drip rate.

$$\frac{\text{Amount of fluid (ml)} \times \text{Drip factor (gtts/ml)}}{\text{Time (minutes)}} = \text{Drip rate (gtts/min)}$$

EXAMPLE 13.1

You are to give dimenhydrinate 50 mg IV. Dimenhydrinate comes in a concentration of 50 mg/ml. You decide to add the dimenhydrinate to a 50-ml bag of normal saline and to administer it over 20 minutes. The drip factor for the tubing is 15.

$$\frac{51 \text{ ml} \times 15 \text{ (gtts/min)}}{20 \text{ min}} = 38.25 \text{ gtts/min}$$

EXAMPLE 13.2

You are caring for a patient who has been admitted with a postoperative wound infection. She has been nauseated and vomiting for the past two days. She has an IV of Ringer's Lactate running at 150 ml/hr. The doctor's order reads *Ancef (cefazolin)*

1 g Q8H IV. The package insert tells you to reconstitute the 1 g vial of Ancef with 2.5 ml of sterile water to give 3 ml of solution. The package insert also says that you can further dilute the Ancef with 50 to 100 ml of Normal Saline, D5W, or Ringer's Lactate. The patient is somewhat dehydrated from the infection and the vomiting, so you decide to put the Ancef in a 100-ml minibag of Ringer's Lactate and to run it over $^1/_2$ an hour. The drip factor for the tubing is 12.

$$\frac{\text{Amount of fluid (ml)} \times \text{Drip factor (gtts/ml)}}{\text{Time (minutes)}} = \text{Drip rate (gtts/min)}$$

$$\frac{103 \text{ ml} \times 12 \text{ gtts/ml}}{30 \text{ min}} = 41.2 \text{ gtts/min}$$

Minibag Used with an IV Pump

A minibag may also be used with an IV pump. Some pumps have a setup similar to that of a gravity IV. The secondary line is attached to a secondary port above the pump. The primary line is clamped off, the pump is reprogrammed for the appropriate flow rate in ml/hr, and the IV medication is administered. Other models have an entry port on the pump itself for a secondary line. The secondary line is attached and the pump is programmed to run this line at the appropriate flow rate in ml/ hr.

Calculation of Flow Rate for Minibags Used with an IV Pump

When calculating the flow rate for a minibag, recall that the time of the infusion is most likely to be in minutes. Since flow rate is in hours, the following formula will allow you to calculate flow rate from minutes:

$$\frac{\text{Amount of solution (ml)}}{\text{Time (minutes)}} \times 60 \text{ (minutes)} = \text{Flow rate}$$

EXAMPLE 13.3

You are to give dimenhydrinate 50 mg IV. Dimenhydrinate comes in a concentration of 50 mg/ml. You decide to add the dimenhydrinate to a 50-ml bag of normal saline and to administer it over 20 minutes.

$$\frac{51 \text{ ml} \times 60}{20} = 153 \text{ ml/hr}$$

You will set the flow rate on the pump for 153 ml/hr.

EXAMPLE 13.4

You are caring for a patient who has been admitted with a postoperative wound infection. She has been nauseated and vomiting for the past two days. She has an IV of Ringer's Lactate running at 150 ml/hr. The doctor's order reads *Ancef (cefazolin) 1 g Q8H IV.* The package insert tells you to reconstitute the 1 g vial of Ancef with 2.5 ml of sterile water to give 3 ml of solution. The package insert also tells you that you can further dilute the Ancef with 50 to 100 ml of normal saline, D5W, or Ringer's Lactate. You decide to put the Ancef in a 100-ml minibag of Ringer's Lactate and to run it over 30 minutes.

$$\frac{103 \text{ ml} \times 60}{30} = 206 \text{ ml/hr}$$

You will set the flow rate on the pump for 206 ml/hr.

IV Soluset

A soluset, also known as a buretrol, volutrol, or pedatrol, is a graduated cylinder that is attached to the IV bag (Figure 13-3). It is used with a gravity IV set and provides both volume control and more accurate control of the speed of administration of fluid or medications. Although it has been largely superseded by IV pumps, it is still used occasionally.

The soluset will hold up to 150 ml of fluid at one time. To fill the soluset, open the air vent clamp and then the bag clamp. The fluid will flow into the soluset. When the required amount of fluid is in the soluset, close the bag clamp. The medication is injected into the medication port, and the soluset gently rotated to mix the medication. Calculate the drip rate and use the tubing clamp to regulate the rate of flow.

Calculation of Drip Rates for Solusets

Solusets have a drip factor of 60, so the drip rate is the same as the flow rate. The flow rate for a soluset is calculated using the same formula as the flow rate for a minibag running on a pump.

$$\frac{\text{Amount of solution (ml)} \times 60}{\text{Time (minutes)}} = \text{Flow rate} = \text{Drip rate}$$

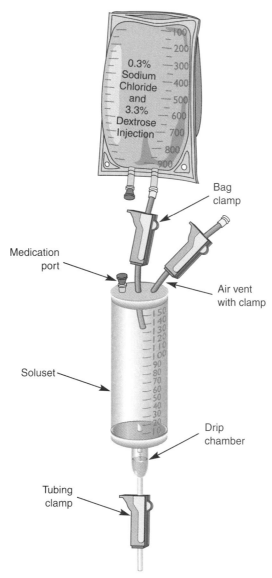

FIGURE 13-3 Soluset attached to IV bag.

EXAMPLE 13.5

The doctor's order reads *furosemide 40 mg IV BID*. The stock is **furosemide 40 mg/4 ml**. Since furosemide is a diuretic and is being administered to help the patient get rid of excess fluid, you want to put the drug in a small volume of fluid. You decide to dilute this so that the patient receives 50 ml of fluid, and you will administer it over 30 minutes.

Add 46 ml of IV solution to the soluset.
Inject 4 ml of furosemide into the soluset to make 50 ml.

$$\frac{\text{Amount of solution (ml)} \times 60}{\text{Time (minutes)}} = \text{Flow rate} = \text{Drip rate}$$

$$\frac{50 \text{ ml} \times 60}{30 \text{ min}} = 100 \text{ ml/hr} = 100 \text{ gtts/min}$$

EXAMPLE 13.6

The doctor's order reads *Zinacef (cefuroxime) 750 mg IV Q8H*. When you reconstitute the stock Zinacef according to the package directions, you have 750 mg of Zinacef in 9 ml of solution. You decide that you will further dilute this so that the patient receives 60 ml of fluid, and you will administer it over 45 minutes.

Add 51 ml of solution to the soluset.
Inject 9 ml of Zinacef into the soluset to make a total of 60 ml.

$$\frac{\text{Amount of solution (ml)} \times 60}{\text{Time (minutes)}} = \text{Flow rate} = \text{Drip rate}$$

$$\frac{60 \text{ ml} \times 60}{45 \text{ min}} = 80 \text{ ml/hr} = 80 \text{ gtts/min}$$

YOU TRY IT

(The answers to these questions are found at the end of the book.)

1. The doctor's order reads *ranitidine 50 mg IV QHS*. The label on the stock reads **ranitidine 50 mg in 2 ml**. You decide that you will further dilute it to 75 ml of fluid and administer it over 20 minutes. What is the drip rate?

2. The doctor's order reads *Solu-Medrol 125 mg IV Q6H*. When reconstituted, the strength is 125 mg/2 ml. You decide that you will further dilute it to 100 ml of fluid and administer it over 40 minutes. What is the drip rate?

3. The doctor's order reads *Kefzol (cefazolin) 1 g IV QID*. When reconstituted, the strength is 125 mg/2 ml. When reconstituted, the strength is 1 g/10 ml. You decide that you will further dilute it to 100 ml of fluid and administer it over 1 hour. What is the drip rate?

4. The doctor's order reads *gentamycin 40 mg IV Q8H*. The label on the stock reads **gentamycin 40 mg in 1 ml**. You decide that you will further dilute it to 50 ml of fluid and administer it over 45 minutes. What is the drip rate?

See full prescribing information for dosage and administration

GENTAMYCIN

40 mg/1 ml

Dispense in a tight, light-resistant container. Store at controlled room temperature 15-30°C.

5. The doctor's order reads *dimenhydrinate 50 mg IV QHS*. The label on the stock reads **dimenhydrinate 50 mg in 1 ml.** You decide that you will further dilute it to 50 ml of fluid and administer it over 20 minutes. What is the drip rate?

Continuous Administration of IV Medications

Some medications are administered continuously for a given period of time. Most of these are highly potent drugs that must be very carefully controlled. They are usually written as weight/hour or weight/min, e.g., *furosemide 2 mg/hr, Dopamine 250 mcg/min,* or *Heparin 900 iu/hr.*

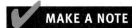 **MAKE A NOTE**

Many of these medications are premixed in an appropriate concentration in an appropriately sized IV bag, but there may be times when you are required to mix one of these bags yourself. These drugs are usually mixed in a small IV bag. To make things simpler for yourself, take the following steps.

Calculate the amount of drug that the patient will receive in 24 hours. For example, if the patient is to receive furosemide at 4 mg/hr, he will get 4 × 24 = 96 mg in 24 hours. Since an IV bag should not hang for more than 24 hours, you want to pre-pare a bag that has approximately this amount of furosemide in it. Now, choose a volume of fluid and an amount of drug that will give you an easily manipulated con-centration or ratio of total drug to total volume of fluid. If you put 100 mg of furosemide in a 100-ml bag of fluid, you will have a concentration of 1 mg : 1 ml. This will make further calculations much simpler.

Calculations for Drugs Ordered as mg/hr

The same methods that are used to calculate other drug dosages (in Unit 3) are used to calculate the rate at which you will run the IV. These drugs should be administered using an IV pump only, so the rate you are calculating will be the flow rate in ml/hr. If you cannot use an IV pump, a gravity IV with microdrip tubing is the next best choice. The drip rate for a microdrip in gtts/min is the same as the flow rate in ml/hr.

EXAMPLE 13.7

The doctor's order reads *diltiazem 10 mg/hr IV for 24 hours*. You follow the package directions to mix your IV minibag and the resulting concentration is 0.83 mg/ml. You must calculate the rate of the IV in ml/hr.

Ratio and Proportion: Means = Extremes

The known ratio is drug (mg) : volume (ml), or 0.83 mg : 1 ml.
The unknown ratio is hourly drug (mg) : hourly volume (ml), or 10 mg : A.

The proportion is 10 mg : A ml = 0.83 mg : 1 ml

$$\downarrow\text{-means-}\downarrow$$
$$10 \text{ mg} : A \text{ ml} = 0.83 \text{ mg} : 1 \text{ ml}$$
$$\uparrow\text{--------extremes---------}\uparrow$$

Means = $0.83 \times A$ = 0.83 A
Extremes = 10×1 = 10

Means = Extremes 0.83A = 10
A = 12
You will run the IV at 12 ml/hr.

Ratio and Proportion: Cross Multiplication of Fractions

When using this method, the ratio is stated in the form of a fraction.

The known ratio is 0.83 mg in 1 ml

This is written $\dfrac{0.83 \text{ (mg)}}{1 \text{ (ml)}}$

The unknown ratio is 10 mg in A ml

This is written $\dfrac{10 \text{ (mg)}}{A \text{ (ml)}}$

Unknown equals known, so these fractions are equal $\dfrac{10 \text{ (mg)}}{A \text{ (ml)}} = \dfrac{0.83 \text{ (mg)}}{1 \text{ (ml)}}$

Cross multiply $\dfrac{10 \text{ mg}}{A \text{ ml}} \nwarrow \nearrow \dfrac{0.83 \text{ mg}}{1 \text{ ml}}$

0.83A = 10 ml
A = 12

Therefore the pump will be set to run at 12 ml/hr.

Formula

$$\frac{\text{Dose } \mathbf{D}\text{esired (mg)}}{\text{Dose on } \mathbf{H}\text{and (mg)}} \times \mathbf{S}\text{tock (ml)} = \mathbf{A}\text{mount (ml) or} \quad \frac{\mathbf{D}}{\mathbf{H}} \times \mathbf{S} = \mathbf{A}$$

Dose **D**esired is 10 mg
Dose on **H**and is 0.83 mg
Stock is 1 ml

$$\frac{\mathbf{D}}{\mathbf{H}} \times \mathbf{S} = \mathbf{A} \qquad \frac{10 \text{ mg}}{0.83 \text{ mg}} \times 1 \text{ (ml)} = A \text{ (ml)}$$

$$\mathbf{A} = 12 \text{ ml}$$

You will set the pump for 12 ml/hr.

Calculations for Drugs Ordered as mcg/min

EXAMPLE 13.8

Some drugs will be ordered in mcg/min rather than mg/hr. You always have to work in the same units, so you will have to convert mcg to mg in order to calculate the dose (ml/min). Further calculation will be required to convert the units to ml/hr so that you can set the pump appropriately.

Doctor's order *dobutamine 100 mcg/min IV for 12 hours*. The dobutamine comes premixed in a concentration of **250 mg/250 ml** or **1 mg/ml**.

Divide by 1,000 to convert mcg to mg 100 mcg = 0.1 mg
The drug will be given at a rate of 0.1 mg/min.
Multiply by 60 to convert minutes to hours: 0.1 mg/min = 6 mg/hr

Ratio and Proportion: Means = Extremes

The known ratio is the concentration or drug (mg) : volume (ml), or 1 mg : 1 ml
The unknown ratio is hourly drug (mg) : hourly volume (ml), or 6 mg : A ml

The proportion is 6 mg : A ml = 1 mg : 1 ml

$$\downarrow\text{-means-}\downarrow$$
$$6 \text{ mg} : A \text{ ml} = 1 \text{ mg} : 1 \text{ ml}$$
$$\uparrow\text{-------extremes------}\uparrow$$

Means = 1 × A = A
Extremes = 6 × 1 = 6
Means = Extremes   A = 6
You will run the IV at 6 ml/hr.

Ratio and Proportion: Cross Multiplication of Fractions

When using this method, the ratio is stated in the form of a fraction.

The known ratio is 1 mg in 1 ml

This is written $\dfrac{1 \text{ (mg)}}{1 \text{ (ml)}}$

The unknown ratio is 6 mg in A ml

This is written $\dfrac{6 \text{ (mg)}}{A \text{ (ml)}}$

Unknown equals known, so these fractions are equal $\dfrac{6 \text{ (mg)}}{A \text{ (ml)}} = \dfrac{1 \text{ (mg)}}{1 \text{ (ml)}}$

Cross multiply $\dfrac{6 \text{ mg}}{A \text{ ml}} \nwarrow\hspace{-1em}\nearrow \dfrac{1 \text{ mg}}{1 \text{ ml}}$

A = 6 ml

Therefore the pump will be set to run at 6 ml/hr.

Formula

$$\frac{\text{Dose } \mathbf{D}\text{esired (mg)}}{\text{Dose on } \mathbf{H}\text{and (mg)}} \times \mathbf{S}\text{tock (ml)} = \mathbf{A}\text{mount (ml)} \quad \text{or} \quad \frac{\mathbf{D}}{\mathbf{H}} \times \mathbf{S} = \mathbf{A}$$

Dose **D**esired is 6 mg
Dose on **H**and is 1 mg
Stock is 1 ml

$$\frac{\mathbf{D}}{\mathbf{H}} \times \mathbf{S} = \mathbf{A} \qquad \frac{6 \text{ mg}}{\cancel{1} \text{ mg}} \times \cancel{1} \text{ (ml)} = A \text{ (ml)}$$

$$\mathbf{A} = 6 \text{ ml}$$

You will set the pump for 6 ml/hr.

Calculations for Drugs Ordered as mcg/kg/min

EXAMPLE 13.9

The order for some of these drugs may be written in mcg/kg/min. The calculations are as follows.

Doctor's order reads *dopamine 3 mcg/kg/min*. You have a stock 250-ml bag of dopamine that has a concentration of **1.6 mg/ml**. The patient weighs **70 kg**.

Calculate the amount of drug/minute. Multiply the dose by the patient's weight.

$$3 \text{ mcg} \times 70 \text{ kg} = 210 \text{ mcg.}$$

The patient will get 210 mcg/minute.

Divide by 1,000 to convert mcg to mg

$$210 \text{ mcg} = 0.21 \text{ mg}$$

The patient will get 0.21 mg/minute.

Multiply by 60 to convert minutes to hours

$$0.21 \text{ mg/min} \times 60 = 12.6 \text{ mg/hr}$$

Ratio and Proportion: Means = Extremes

The known ratio is drug (mg) : volume (ml), or 1.6 mg : 1 ml
The unknown ratio is hourly drug (mg) : hourly volume (ml), or 12.6 mg : A

The proportion is 12.6 mg : A ml = 1.6 mg : 1 ml

$$\downarrow\text{-means-}\downarrow$$
$$12.6 \text{ mg} : A \text{ ml} = 1.6 \text{ mg} : 1 \text{ ml}$$
$$\uparrow\text{---------extremes----------}\uparrow$$

Means = $1.6 \times A = 1.6$ A
Extremes = $12.6 \times 1 = 12.6$
Means = Extremes   1.6 A = 12.6
A = 7.8

The pump requires you to enter a whole number, so you will run the IV at 8 ml/hr.

Ratio and Proportion: Cross Multiplication of Fractions

When using this method, the ratio is stated in the form of a fraction.

The known ratio is 1.6 mg in 1 ml

This is written $\dfrac{1.6 \text{ (mg)}}{1 \text{ (ml)}}$

The unknown ratio is 12.6 mg in A ml

This is written $\dfrac{12.6 \text{ (mg)}}{A \text{ (ml)}}$

Unknown equals known, so these fractions are equal $\dfrac{12.6 \text{ (mg)}}{A \text{ (ml)}} = \dfrac{1.6 \text{ (mg)}}{1 \text{ (ml)}}$

Cross multiply $\dfrac{12.6 \text{ mg}}{\text{A ml}} \quad \dfrac{1.6 \text{ mg}}{1 \text{ ml}}$

1.6A = 12.6 ml
A = 7.8

Therefore the pump will be set to run at 8 ml/hr.

Formula

$$\dfrac{\text{Dose Desired (mg)}}{\text{Dose on Hand (mg)}} \times \text{Stock (ml)} = \text{Amount (ml)} \quad \text{or} \quad \dfrac{D}{H} \times S = A$$

Dose Desired is 12.6 mg
Dose on Hand is 1.6 mg
Stock is 1 ml

$$\dfrac{D}{H} \times S = A \qquad \dfrac{12.6 \text{ mg}}{1.6 \text{ mg}} \times 1 \text{ (ml)} = A \text{ (ml)}$$

$$A = 7.8 \text{ ml}$$

You will set the pump for 8 ml/hr.

YOU TRY IT

(The answers to these questions are found at the end of the book.)

1. Doctor's order reads *furosemide 4 mg/hr IV*. The bag we have mixed has a concentration of furosemide **100 mg/100 ml** of IV fluid. At what flow rate will you run the pump?

2. Doctor's order reads *lidocaine 2 mg/min IV*. Lidocaine comes in a premixed 250-ml bag with a concentration of 8 mg/ml. At what flow rate will you run the pump?

3. Doctor's order reads *Isuprel (isoproterenol) 5 mcg/min IV*. Manufacturer's directions state that 1 mg of Isuprel is to be added to a 250 ml bag of D5W. At what flow rate will you run the pump?

ISOPROTERENOL

See full prescribing information for dosage and administration

Manufacturer's Directions:

1 mg of isuprel is to be added to a **250-ml** bag of **D5W**

Dispense in a tight, light-resistant container. Store at controlled room temperature 15-30°C.

4. Doctor's order reads *nitroglycerine 400 mcg/min IV*. The premixed bag contains a concentration of 0.2 mg/ml. At what flow rate will you run the pump?

5. Doctor's order reads *dobutamine 5 mcg/kg/min IV for 6 hours*. The bag of dobutamine has a concentration of 1 mg/ml. The patient weighs 55 kg. At what flow rate will you run the pump?

Portable Continuous Infusion Pumps

There are situations in which the patient needs parenteral medications on a continuous basis over an extended period of time. In order to facilitate this, small, specialized pumps have been developed that can deliver medications into either a vein or subcutaneous tissue (Figure 13-4).

One of the common uses for portable continuous infusion pumps is to provide continuous analgesia for patients with chronic or terminal pain. The pump delivers a small amount of analgesia all the time. It can also be programmed to allow the patient to administer a bolus dose when his pain level increases. The use of continuous infusion for analgesia has a number of advantages for the patient. It requires less drug to maintain analgesia than it does to decrease high levels of pain. Allowing the patient to self-medicate gives him some control over his condition, and usually results in the use of less, rather than more drug. The pumps are small enough that they can be put in a pocket or clipped to a belt. This gives patients increased mobility and independence and allows them to have a more normal lifestyle.

The other common use for portable continuous infusion pumps is for the continuous subcutaneous administration of insulin. (See Chapter 14.)

Portable continuous infusion pumps have a reservoir for the drug. Most pumps use preloaded cassettes of medication, although a few older pumps require that the nurse fill the reservoir with specific amounts of drug and normal saline to achieve a given concentration. Each manufacturer has different instructions for programming the pumps and the directions must be followed very carefully in order to deliver the appropriate amount of drug.

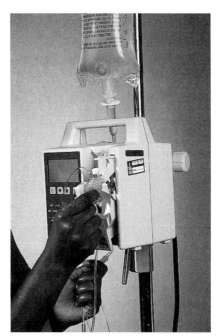

FIGURE 13-4 Portable continuous infusion pump. (From Taylor, C., Lillis, C., & LeMone, P. [2004]. *Photo Atlas of Medication Administration.* [p. 46]. Philadelphia: Lippincott Williams & Wilkins.)

Self Test

Answers to these questions are found at the end of the book.

Calculate the drip rate for the following IV medications. The medications are added to a minibag which is used with a gravity IV.

1. Doctor's order reads *metronidazole 100 mg IV Q8H*. The metronidazole comes premixed in a 100-ml minibag and is to be administered over 45 minutes. The drip factor is 12.

2. Doctor's order reads *Lasix (furosemide) 40 mg IV stat*. The label on the vial reads **Lasix 40 mg/4 ml**. You decide to mix the Lasix in a 50-ml bag and administer it over 20 minutes. The drip factor is 15.

FUROSEMIDE

See full prescribing information for dosage and administration

40 mg/4 ml

Dispense in a tight, light-resistant container. Store at controlled room temperature 15-30°C.

3. Doctor's order reads *Rocephin 1 g IV Q12H*. When reconstituted, there is 1 g of Rocephin in 10 ml of solution. You decide to dilute it in a 100 ml bag of normal saline and administer it over 1 hour. The drip factor is 15.

See full prescribing information for dosage and administration

ROCEPHIN

40 mg/ml

Dispense in a tight, light-resistant container. Store at controlled room temperature 15-30°C.

4. Doctor's order reads *Zinacef 1.5 g IV Q8H*. When reconstituted, there is 1.5 g of Zinacef in 16 ml of solution. You decide to dilute it in 50 ml of normal saline and administer it over 30 minutes. The drip factor is 10.

5. Doctor's order reads *ranitidine 50 mg IV QHS*. The ranitidine is in a vial labelled 25 mg/ml. You decide to dilute it in 50 ml of normal saline and administer it over 25 minutes. The drip factor is 15.

Calculate the flow rate for the following IV medications. The medications are added to a minibag and administered using an IV pump.

6. Doctor's order reads *Cipro (ciprofloxacin) 400 mg IV Q12H*. Cipro must be diluted in 250 ml of normal saline. You decide to administer it over 90 minutes.

7. Doctor's order reads *Pantoloc (pantoprazole) 40 mg IV QHS*. When reconstituted, there are 40 mg of Pantoloc in 10 ml of solution. It should be further diluted in 100 ml of normal saline and administered over 1 hour.

8. Doctor's order reads *Solu-Medrol (methylprednisolone) 500 mg IV Q8H*. When reconstituted, there are 500 mg of Solu-Medrol in 8 ml of solution. You decide to dilute it in 50 ml of normal saline and administer it over 30 minutes.

9. Doctor's order reads *vancomycin 1 g IV Q8H*. When reconstituted there is 1 g of vancomycin in 20 ml of solution. This must be further diluted in 250 ml of normal saline and administered over 60 minutes.

10. Doctor's order reads *Ancef (cefazolin) 1 g IV Q8H*. When reconstituted there is 1 g of Ancef in 3 ml of solution. You decide to dilute it in 50 ml of normal saline and administer it over 20 minutes.

Calculate the drip rate for the following IV medications. The medications are added to a soluset.

11. Doctor's order reads *gentamycin 40 mg IV Q8H*. Gentamycin is supplied in a concentration of 40 mg/ml. You decide to further dilute it to 125 ml of fluid and to administer it over 90 minutes.

See full prescribing information for dosage and administration

GENTAMYCIN

40 mg/ml

Dispense in a tight, light-resistant container. Store at controlled room temperature 15-30°C.

12. Doctor's order reads *clindamycin 600 mg IV Q6H*. Clindamycin is supplied in 4-ml vials that have a strength of 150 mg/ml. The package states that you should further dilute it to 50 ml of compatible IV solution and administer it over 20 minutes.

13. Doctor's order reads *Rocephin (ceftriaxone) 1 g IV Q12H.* When reconstituted, there is 1 g of Rocephin in 10 ml of solution. You decide to further dilute it to 75 ml of fluid and administer it over 45 minutes.

14. Doctor's order reads *Cefizox (ceftizoxime) 2 g IV Q12H.* When reconstituted, there are 2 g of Cefizox in 20 ml of solution. You decide to further dilute it to 70 ml of fluid and administer it over 75 minutes.

15. Doctor's order reads *dimenhydrinate 50 mg IV Q4H PRN for nausea.* Dimenhydrinate is supplied in a concentration of 50 mg/ml. You decide to further dilute it to 30 ml of fluid and to administer it over 15 minutes.

Calculate the flow rate for the following medications administered using an IV pump.

16. Doctor's order reads *magnesium sulphate IV 1 g/hour × 24 hours.* Your drug guide tells you to mix 25 g of magnesium sulphate in 250 ml of D5W.

17. Doctor's order reads *Pantoloc (pantoprazole) IV 8 mg/hour*. Pharmacy sends you a 100 ml bag which has a concentration of 0.4 mg/ml.

18. Doctor's order reads *amiodarone IV 1 mg/min*. Hospital policy states that you will mix 450 mg of amiodarone in 250 ml of D5W.

19. Doctor's order reads *amiodarone IV 15 mg/min for 10 min for breakthrough arrhythmia*. Hospital policy states that you will mix 450 mg of amiodarone in 250 ml of D5W.

20. Doctor's order reads *theophylline IV 0.5 mg/kg/hr*. Theophylline comes in a pre-mixed bag of 500 mg/500 ml of D5W. The patient's weight is 68 kg.

Special Calculations

150 mg: A ml: 50 mg: 2 ml

(g/ml)

75 mg: A ml: 100 mg: 1 ml

Preparation and Administration of Insulin

The student will:

- describe the different preparations of insulin
- identify the appropriate syringe to be used to draw up insulin
- describe the correct procedure for drawing up one or more types of insulin in the same syringe
- interpret a titrated/sliding scale insulin order correctly
- describe the correct procedure for administering insulin intravenously
- describe the insulin delivery devices
- identify the elements of appropriate charting associated with administration of insulin

Insulin dependent diabetes mellitus (IDDM), type 1 diabetes: disease process in which there is a complete absence of endogenous insulin production.

Noninsulin-dependent diabetes mellitus (NIDDM), Type 2 diabetes: disease process in which there is insufficient endogenous insulin production and/or cellular resistance to the action of insulin.

Endogenous insulin: insulin produced by the patient's pancreas.

Exogenous insulin: insulin produced outside the patient's body and administered as a medication.

Onset: the time when a dose of insulin begins to act.

Peak: the period of time when a dose of insulin is most active.

Duration: the total length of time that a dose of insulin is active.

Titration: the process of changing the amount of a medication by small increments until a desired result is achieved.

Insulin is a hormone produced by the beta cells of the pancreas in response to an increase in the amount of glucose in the blood. The role of insulin is to actively transport the glucose from the blood stream into the cells. The use of exogenous insulin in the treatment of diabetes mellitus was discovered and developed in Canada.

Diabetes mellitus is a disorder of carbohydrate metabolism in which the patient is unable to move sufficient glucose from the vascular system to the cells. There are several different types of diabetes mellitus. Insulin-dependent diabetes mellitus (IDDM), or Type 1 diabetes, is characterized by a complete absence of endogenous insulin production. These patients must be given exogenous insulin in order to sustain life. Noninsulin-dependent diabetes mellitus (NIDDM), or Type 2 diabetes, is characterized by insufficient endogenous insulin production and cellular resistance to the action of insulin. These patients may be treated with oral hypoglycemic drugs; despite the name of the disorder, they may require treatment with exogenous insulin. Gestational diabetes occurs in the 2nd and 3rd trimesters of pregnancy. At this point in the pregnancy, there may be both insufficient insulin and increased cellular resistance to the action of insulin in the mother. Gestational diabetes is also treated with exogenous insulin.

Insulin is digested in the gastrointestinal tract when taken orally, so it must be given parenterally. The usual routes for insulin administration are subcutaneous and intravenous. Insulin is almost never given intramuscularly.

Insulin Preparations

When insulin was first used to treat diabetes, it was extracted from the pancreas of cows or pigs. While beef and pork insulin are similar to human insulin, there are some slight differences. These differences are sufficient to cause adverse effects in a number of patients. Recently it has become possible to use biotechnology to manufacture insulin that is identical to human insulin. Most patients use the bioengineered human type insulin, but a small amount of beef and pork insulin are still available for older patients who do not wish to change drugs.

Insulin that is identical to endogenous insulin (regular insulin) is fairly rapidly absorbed from subcutaneous tissue. It begins to act (onset) in 30 minutes, is most effective (peak) in 2–4 hours and is active (duration) for 5–7 hours. Use of regular insulin means that a patient would need several injections daily to maintain blood sugar at appropriate levels. Various modifications have been made to regular insulin so that the onset, peak, and duration are different. Table 14-1 identifies some of the most common preparations of insulin.

Insulin Syringes

The amount of insulin to be administered is identified in units. (See Chapter 4 for a definition and description of units.) Most insulin is manufactured with 100 units/ml (u/ml or U100). Insulin is drawn up in a specialized syringe called an insulin syringe (Figure 14-1). Insulin should not be drawn up in any other kind of syringe, and these syringes should only be used for insulin. The syringe and its package are clearly marked as U100. This should always be compared to the bottle of insulin, which will be marked with the strength of the insulin. The side of the syringe is marked so that the dosage can be measured very accurately.

Insulin syringes are similar in size and appearance to tuberculin syringes but they are not interchangeable. Insulin syringes have a finer gauge needle and the graduations along the side are marked in units/ml. The graduations along the side of a tuberculin syringe are marked in 1/100 of a ml. Tuberculin syringes have a differently shaped hub

TABLE 14-1
COMMON PREPARATIONS OF INSULIN

Preparation	Description	Onset	Peak	Duration
Ultra Short-Acting Insulin: lispro insulin Humalog	Clear, biosynthetic insulin that has been modified for very rapid absorption and onset of action.	15 min	45 min–2$\frac{1}{2}$ hr	3–4 hr
Short-Acting Insulin: regular insulin Toronto insulin Humulin R	Clear, biosynthetic insulin that is identical to human endogenous insulin.	30 min	2–4 hr	5–7 hr
Intermediate-Acting Insulin: NPH Novolin ge NPH Humulin N	Cloudy, biosynthetic insulin. Zinc and protamine have been added to delay absorption and prolong the action of the insulin.	1$\frac{1}{2}$ hr	4–12 hr	24 hr
Intermediate-Acting Insulin: Lente Novolin ge Lente Humulin L	Cloudy, biosynthetic insulin. Zinc has been added to delay absorption and prolong the action of the insulin.	2$\frac{1}{2}$ hr	7–15 hr	22 hr
Mixed Insulin:	Premixed solution of regular insulin and NPH insulin in a fixed ratio.			
Novolin ge 20/80	1 ml of 20/80 contains 20 units of regular insulin and 80 units of NPH insulin.	30 min	2–12 hr	24 hr
Novolin ge 30/70	1 ml of 30/70 contains 30 units of regular insulin and 80 units of NPH insulin.	30 min	2–12 hr	24 hr

at the base of the needle (Figure 14-2). There is approximately 0.05 ml of air in the "dead space" of the hub of the needle. When used for insulin, 5 units of insulin occupy that space. If two kinds of insulin are drawn up in one syringe, you will end up with an extra 5 units of the one drawn up first, while 5 units of the second kind are trapped in the hub. When you are working with small doses of insulin, 5 units can represent a significant proportion of the dose.

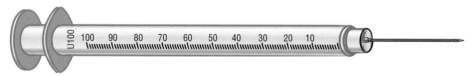

FIGURE 14-1 Insulin syringe.

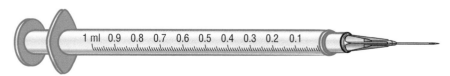

FIGURE 14-2 Tuberculin syringe.

KEEP IT SAFE While almost all of the insulin used today is prepared as 100 u/ml, other strengths are available. Higher concentrations of insulin may be found in hospital pharmacies where they are used to prepare IV infusions of insulin. In the past, insulin was manufactured with a strength of 40 u/ml and 80 u/ml. U40 and U80 syringes were also available.

The likelihood of encountering these is very small, but it is important that you always check to ensure that both the insulin and the syringe are the same.

Preparing Insulin for Subcutaneous Injection

Insulin is usually administered subcutaneously. If it is injected intramuscularly, the rate of absorption is usually increased, but it is also unpredictable because it varies with the amount of blood flow to the muscle. Flexing the muscle after injection causes more rapid absorption.

Insulin is stored in vials, and when a single type of insulin is drawn up, the procedure is the same as for any injection from a vial.

Frequently, the best control of diabetes is achieved with a mixture of regular insulin and one of the intermediate-acting insulins. Premixed insulin may be ordered, e.g., *Novolin 30/70 42 u QAM*. In this case, 42 units of insulin will be drawn up from the appropriate premixed vial. The physician may, however, order two different insulins to be given at the same time, e.g., *Regular insulin 18 u QAM and NPH insulin 33 u QAM*. The following procedure is used to draw up the two insulins in the same syringe. This procedure is very similar to that for drawing up any two medications from two vials. (See Chapter 11.) Since the regular insulin is clear and the intermediate insulins are cloudy in appearance, it is usual to refer to them as *clear* and *cloudy*.

- Calculate the total volume of insulin to be drawn up, e.g., 18 *u* + 33 *u* = 51 *u*.
- Roll the cloudy insulin gently between your palms so that the solution is well mixed. Do not shake insulin; the molecules are large and fragile.
- Clean the top of each vial with an alcohol swab to remove surface dust or debris.
- Draw up an amount of air equal to the dose of *cloudy* insulin and inject it into the cloudy bottle. Make sure that the tip of the needle does not touch the solution.
- Draw up an amount of air equal to the dose of *clear* insulin and inject it into the clear bottle, e.g., *18 u* (Figure 14-3).
- Withdraw the appropriate dose of insulin from the *clear* bottle.
- Insert the needle into the *cloudy* bottle and pull back on the plunger until the syringe is filled with the amount equal to the total calculated above, e.g., *51 u* (Figure 14-4).

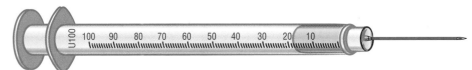

FIGURE 14-3 18 units of insulin.

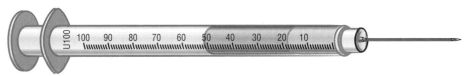

FIGURE 14-4 51 units of insulin.

KEEP IT SAFE It is important that the short-acting, regular or clear insulin be drawn up first. This is to prevent contamination of the regular insulin by the intermediate or cloudy insulin in the syringe. Regular insulin is the only insulin that can be given intravenously. Contamination of a vial of regular insulin may not be visible, but it may be dangerous to the patient if the vial is subsequently used for intravenous administration.

YOU TRY IT

(The answers to these questions are found at the end of the book.)

On the following insulin syringes, mark the amount of regular insulin and the total amount of insulin prescribed in the following doctor's orders.

1. *Regular insulin 17 u and NPH insulin 28 u.*

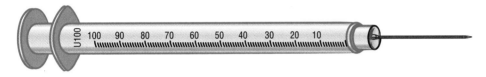

2. *Regular insulin 9 u and NPH insulin 22 u.*

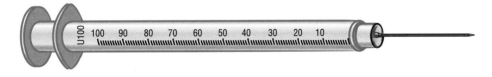

3. *Regular insulin 20 u and NPH insulin 44 u.*

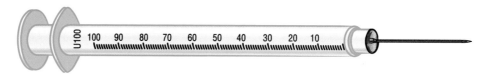

4. *Regular insulin 12 u and NPH insulin 37 u.*

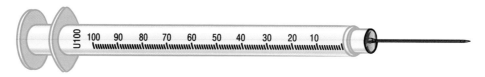

5. *Regular insulin 5 u and NPH insulin 16 u.*

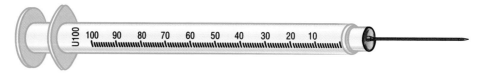

Titrated Insulin

Some insulin orders are titrated by blood sugar. The patient's blood sugar is identified using a hand-held glucometer, and the amount of insulin to be given varies with the amount of sugar. This is also called sliding scale insulin, insulin by reaction, or insulin by glucometer. For example, the doctor's order reads:

Regular insulin sc by glucometer TID AC and HS
  blood sugar   *0–9.9 no insulin*
                10.0–14.9 give 6 units
                15.0–19.9 give 8 units
                20.0–24.9 give 10 units

YOU TRY IT

(The answers to these questions are found at the end of the book.)

Using the above doctor's order, how much insulin will you give in the following situations?

1. At 0730 hrs your patient's blood sugar is 8.4.

2. At 1130 hrs your patient's blood sugar is 17.0.

3. At 1730 hrs your patient's blood sugar is 13.7.

4. At 2200 hrs your patient's blood sugar is 12.5.

Intravenous Insulin

For most patients who require insulin, subcutaneous injection is the route of choice. There are, however, some situations in which it is preferable to administer insulin intravenously. These are usually situations in which either very rapid response or continuous administration is required. Only regular insulin can be administered intravenously.

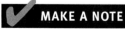

MAKE A NOTE

Some older text books and hospital policy manuals state that clear insulin may be given IV but cloudy insulin may not. This used to be appropriate in the past, but the development of the clear, ultra short-acting insulins means that you cannot rely on this rule of thumb any more. Only regular insulin can be given IV.

Regular insulin is usually diluted in a minibag and administered continuously. It is normally diluted in a solution of 1 unit per 1 or 2 ml. The most common dilution is 125 units of regular insulin in 250 ml of normal saline. The doctor's order will identify the number of units per hour, e.g., *insulin IV 8 units/ hour*. Calculation of the rate is the same as for medications ordered in mg/hr. (See Chapter 12 for the calculation method.)

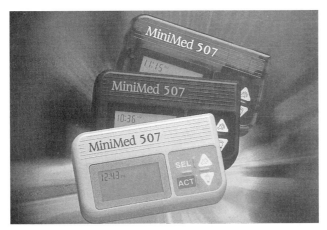

FIGURE 14-5 MiniMed insulin pump. (From Evans-Smith, P. (2005). *Taylor's clinical nursing skills: A nursing approach* [p. 183]. Philadelphia: Lippincott Williams & Wilkins, 2005.)

Insulin Delivery Devices

Diabetes is a chronic disease that ultimately must be managed by the patient. Recently, two kinds of insulin delivery devices have been developed to make diabetes management easier.

Insulin Pens

Insulin pens are an alternative to a syringe. A cartridge of insulin is loaded into the pen. A dial on the pen is set to the number of units desired. The pen is placed against the injection site and a button is pushed. This activates a small needle that penetrates the skin, and the required dose of insulin is injected. Pens may be used to deliver any of the usual types of insulin. Most pens use a 3-ml cartridge of U-100 insulin. This lasts for several days for most patients. The pen does not require refrigeration during that time.

Many patients find the pen easier to manipulate than a syringe, and it is easier to set a dial accurately than to get exactly the right amount into the syringe.

Insulin Pumps

An insulin pump is a mechanical reservoir and pump (Figure 14-5) that is connected by a short piece of tubing to a subcutaneous needle inserted into the patient's abdomen. It is loaded with 2 to 3 ml of ultra-fast-acting or regular insulin. There is a continuous subcutaneous infusion of insulin to cover the basal rate of glucose metabolism. It also allows for bolus doses to provide the appropriate amount of insulin required for each meal of the day. The patient checks his blood sugar before a meal, calculates the amount of carbohydrate he or she is planning to eat and administers the appropriate amount of insulin to metabolize the carbohydrates. Insulin pumps, when combined with frequent glucose monitoring, can provide more precise control of blood sugar than the other methods of delivery.

Init	Signature
AC	Anita Cortez RN
KD	Ken Doyle RN

AGH
Anywhere General Hospital
DIABETIC
RECORD

3764092
Hailley, Isaac
442 Mill St
Anywhere,
Ontario

Allergies   ASA

Diagnosis   IDDM
Coronary Artery Disease

Date Time	Glucometer	Insulin by Reaction	Scheduled Insulin	Init
24/04/05 0730	7.8		NPH 22 u sc	AC
1130	11.2	Regular insulin 6 u sc		AC
1630	12.4	Regular insulin 6 u sc	NPH 18 u sc	KD
2200	6.3			KD

FIGURE 14-6 Sample diabetic record.

The insulin pump requires the patient to make a high degree of commitment to diabetes control. It is also the most expensive of the insulin delivery devices.

Documentation of Insulin Administration

Insulin administration must, of course, be documented. In addition to the usual medication charting, it is also important to chart the glucometer reading at the time of administration. This allows for manipulation of the amount of insulin to maintain blood sugars at optimum levels. Some institutions have specialized forms for the documentation of glucometer and insulin (Figure 14-6). If there is no specialized form, the glucometer reading should be added to the MAR or, if that is not possible, **recorded** in the nursing progress notes.

chapter 14

Self Test

Answers to these questions are found at the end of the book.

Mrs. Evelyn Maracle is a 57-year-old woman who has been recently diagnosed with NIDDM or Type 2 diabetes mellitus. She has been reluctant to accept this diagnosis and admits to being noncompliant with her diet. She has been admitted to your hospital floor with a blood sugar of 39 mmol/L. Her doctor's orders are as follows.

Insulin IV 12 u/hr until 0700 hrs tomorrow.
NPH insulin 22 u sc $\frac{1}{2}$ hr ac breakfast
NPH insulin 16 u sc $\frac{1}{2}$ ac supper
Glucometer TID $\frac{1}{2}$ hr ac meals and HS

    Glucometer   *< 9.9 no insulin*
                          10.0–12.9 give 6 units regular insulin
                          13.0–15.9 give 9 units regular insulin
                          16.0–18.9 give 11 units regular insulin
                          19.0–21.9 give 13 units regular insulin
                          > 22 call for further orders

The IV insulin is in a premixed bag with a strength of 125 u of insulin in 250 ml of NS. Hospital policy in your institution states that IV insulin is always administered using a pump.

1. At what rate will you run the IV?

2. Mrs. Maracle's glucometer readings have been recorded on the diabetic record (Figure 14-7). Using those readings, document all of the insulin that should be administered over the next two days.

Init	Signature	**AGH** Anywhere General Hospital DIABETIC RECORD	5723753 Maracle, Evelyn 546 Front St. Apt. 448 Anywhere, Ontario

Allergies   *NKA*

Diagnosis *NIDDM*
Arterial Insufficiency

Date Time	Glucometer	Insulin by Reaction	Scheduled Insulin	Init
06/10/04 *0730*	*14.7*			
1130	*10.2*			
1630	*16.3*			
2200	*7.1*			
07/10/04 *0730*	*19.4*			
1130	*12.3*			
1630	*14.1*			
2200	*8.8*			

FIGURE 14-7 Mrs. Maracle's diabetic record.

3.   On the syringes below, identify the time and amounts of each mixed insulin that should be given as a result of the above doctor's orders and glucometer readings.

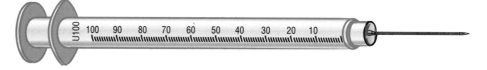

Time _____

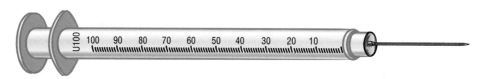

Time _____

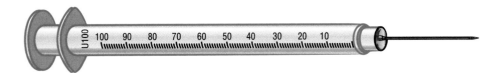

Time _____

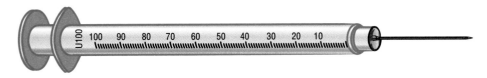

Time _____

Anticoagulant Therapy

The student will:

- **describe heparin**

- **describe the assessment and evaluation associated with anticoagulant therapy**

- **describe the appropriate procedure for preparing and administering subcutaneous heparin**

- **calculate subcutaneous doses of heparin correctly**

- **describe the appropriate procedure for preparing and administering intravenous heparin therapy**

- **calculate intravenous doses of heparin correctly**

- **describe low molecular weight heparins**

- **describe oral anticoagulant (warfarin) therapy**

Clotting mechanism: process by which inactive circulating coagulation factors are activated to convert prothrombin to thrombin and fibrinogen to fibrin, creating a fibrin clot.

Intrinsic pathway: activation of the clotting mechanism by injury to the endothelium of a blood vessel (surface agent). Proceeds slowly.

Extrinsic pathway: activation of the clotting mechanism by tissue injury (tissue factor). Proceeds quickly.

Common pathway: the end stage of the clotting mechanism. It can be activated by either the intrinsic or the extrinsic pathway.

Thrombolytic: substance that causes the breakdown of a fibrin clot.

Activated partial thromboplastin time (APTT): surface active agent is added to plasma and the time it takes to form a clot is measured. Used to evaluate the intrinsic and common pathways and monitor heparin therapy.

Prothrombin time (PT): tissue factor is added to plasma and the time it takes for a clot to form is measured. Used to evaluate the extrinsic and common pathways and monitor warfarin/coumarin therapy.

International normalized ratio (INR): international agreement on norms for prothrombin time.

Anticoagulants are used to interfere with some aspect of the clotting mechanism. They are used prophylactically to prevent the development of blood clots in patients who are at risk for inappropriate clotting. Patients who are immobile, those who have recently had some types of vascular, urologic, gynecologic or orthopaedic surgery, and some pregnant women are at risk for the development of deep-vein thrombosis. Patients with a mechanical heart valve prosthesis require prophylactic anticoagulants because these devices tend to generate clots. Anticoagulants are also used prophylactically to decrease clotting in patients with atrial fibrillation, severe unstable angina, and acute myocardial infarction. There are situations blood is removed from the body and then returned to it such as blood transfusions, hemodialysis, and cardiopulmonary bypass. Anticoagulants are used to keep the blood from clotting while it is outside the body. Diagnostic tests requiring unclotted blood will be collected in tubes containing a small amount of an anticoagulant.

Larger doses of anticoagulants are also used therapeutically. If an inappropriate clot such as a deep-vein thrombosis or pulmonary embolus forms, anticoagulants will prevent extension or enlargement of the clot until the body's fibrinolytic system breaks down the clot. There are a variety of drugs that alter the clotting mechanism. In this chapter we will deal with three types of anticoagulants: heparin, low molecular weight heparins, and warfarin.

Heparin

Heparin is a natural substance that is produced by the mast cells of the liver and by basophil leukocytes. It interferes with the intrinsic and common pathways of the clotting mechanism. It also contributes to the breakdown of existing clots by interfering with extension of the clot. This allows natural thrombolytics to act more effectively. The relationship between the dose of heparin and its effectiveness is not linear, so ongoing monitoring is an important part of heparin therapy. Heparin therapy is monitored by measuring APTT (activated partial thromboplastin time).

Because it is not absorbed through the GI mucosa, heparin is administered either subcutaneously or intravenously. It is not given intramuscularly due to the risk of extensive bleeding into the muscle at the injection site. Heparin is measured in units and is available in a variety of strengths of preparation.

Subcutaneous Administration

Heparin is used prophylactically to prevent thromboemboli in patients who have had certain types of surgery and/or who are immobilized. When used in this way, it is usually administered subcutaneously. The strength of the solution is 10 000 u/ml and the usual dose is 2 500 to 7 500 u. This means that the amount to be administered is a fraction of a millilitre. The most accurate syringe for this amount of medication is a tuberculin syringe (see below), which is marked in 1/100th of a millilitre.

The needle should be 27 gauge or smaller and 1/2″ long. The usual methods for calculating the amount of medication are used to calculate the amount of heparin.

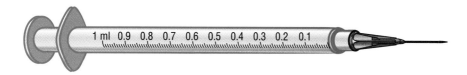

EXAMPLE 15.1

The doctor's order reads *heparin 6 000 u sc bid*. The label on the ampoule of heparin reads **Heparin 10 000 u/ml.**

Ratio and Proportion: Means = Extremes

The known ratio is 10 000 u : 1 ml
The unknown ratio is 6 000 u : A ml

The proportion is 6 000 u : A ml = 10 000 u : 1 ml

$$\downarrow\text{-means-}\downarrow$$
$$6\ 000\ u : A\ ml = 10\ 000\ u : 1\ ml$$
$$\uparrow\text{--------extremes-----------}\uparrow$$

Means = 10 000 $\times$ A = 10 000A
Extremes = 6 000 $\times$ 1 = 6 000

Means = Extremes   10 000A = 6 000
Divide both by 10 000
A = 0.6 ml
You will give 0.6 ml of Heparin.

Ratio and Proportion: Cross Multiplication of Fractions

When using this method, the ratio is stated in the form of a fraction.

The known ratio is 10 000 u in 1 ml

This is written $\dfrac{10\ 000\ (u)}{1\ (ml)}$

The unknown ratio is 6 000 in A ml

This is written $\dfrac{6\ 000\ u}{A\ (ml)}$

Unknown equals known, so these fractions are equal $\dfrac{6\ 000\ (u)}{A\ (ml)} = \dfrac{10\ 000\ (u)}{1\ (ml)}$

Cross multiply $\dfrac{6\ 000\ u}{A\ ml} \diagup\!\!\!\!\diagdown \dfrac{10\ 000\ u}{1\ ml}$

10 000A = 6 000, or A = 0.6 ml

Therefore the dose to be given is 0.6 ml.

Formula

$$\frac{\text{Dose \textbf{D}esired (u)}}{\text{Dose on \textbf{H}and (u)}} \times \textbf{S}\text{tock (ml)} = \textbf{A}\text{mount (ml)} \quad \text{or} \quad \frac{\textbf{D}}{\textbf{H}} \times \textbf{S} = \textbf{A}$$

Dose **D**esired is 6 000 u
Dose on **H**and is 10 000 u
Stock is 2 ml

$$\frac{D}{H} \times S = A \qquad\qquad \frac{6\ 000\ u}{10\ 000\ u} \times 1\ (ml) = A\ (ml)$$

A = 0.6 ml

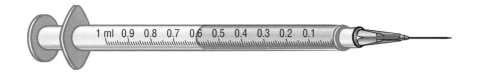

YOU TRY IT

(The answers to these questions are found at the end of the book.)

The label on the vial of heparin reads **heparin 10 000 u/ml.** How much heparin will you draw up for each of the following doctor's orders?

1. *Heparin 5 000 u sc bid.*

2. *Heparin 2 500 u sc qid.*

3. *Heparin 4 000 u sc bid.*

4. *Heparin 5 500 u sc bid.*

Intravenous Administration

Heparin is used therapeutically to treat a number of different problems. Probably the most common therapeutic use is to treat thromboemboli, or blood clots, within the vascular system. The standard concentration of IV heparin in this situation is 25 000 u of heparin in 250 ml of normal saline. Heparin binds to a variety of proteins in the blood, so the dose that will achieve the desired result is somewhat variable. The goal for therapeutic heparin is to raise the APPT to 1.5–2.5 times the control or normal value. Doctor's orders for IV heparin are usually written as the number of units per hour (u/hr), or the number of units per kilogram per hour (u/kg/hr). These rates are calculated using the same method as other IV drug orders that are written in this way. (See Chapter 13.)

EXAMPLE 15.2

Doctor's order reads *heparin IV 800 u/hr.* The heparin is in the standard concentration of 25 000 u/250 ml NS. This gives a concentration of 100 u/ml.

Ratio and Proportion: Means = Extremes

The known ratio is the concentration or drug (u) : volume (ml) or 100 u : 1 ml.
The unknown ratio is hourly drug (u) : hourly volume (ml) or 800 u : A.
The proportion is 800 u : A ml = 100 u : 1 ml.

$$\downarrow\text{-means-}\downarrow$$
$$800 \text{ u} : A \text{ ml} = 100 \text{ u} : 1 \text{ ml}$$
$$\uparrow\text{--------extremes---------}\uparrow$$

Means = 100 × A = 100A
Extremes = 800 × 1 = 800
Means = Extremes 100A = 800
A = 8 ml/hr
You will run the IV at 8 ml/hr.

Ratio and Proportion: Cross Multiplication of Fractions

When using this method, the ratio is stated in the form of a fraction.
The known ratio is 100 u in 1 ml

This is written $\dfrac{100 \text{ (u)}}{1 \text{ (ml)}}$

The unknown ratio is 800 u in A ml

This is written $\dfrac{800 \,(\text{u})}{A \,(\text{ml})}$

Unknown equals known, so these fractions are equal $\dfrac{800 \,(\text{u})}{A \,(\text{ml})} = \dfrac{100 \,(\text{u})}{1 \,(\text{ml})}$

Cross multiply $\dfrac{800 \,(\text{u})}{A \,(\text{ml})} \nwarrow \nearrow \dfrac{100 \,(\text{u})}{1 \,(\text{ml})}$

100A = 800 ml
A = 8
Therefore the pump will be set to run at 8 ml/hr.

Formula

$$\frac{\text{Dose } \textbf{D}\text{esired (u)}}{\text{Dose on } \textbf{H}\text{and (u)}} \times \textbf{S}\text{tock (ml)} = \textbf{A}\text{mount (ml)} \quad \text{or} \quad \frac{\textbf{D}}{\textbf{H}} \times \textbf{S} = \textbf{A}$$

Dose **D**esired is 800 u
Dose on **H**and is 100 u
Stock is 1 ml

$$\frac{\textbf{D}}{\textbf{H}} \times \textbf{S} = \textbf{A} \qquad\qquad \frac{800 \text{ u}}{100 \text{ u}} \times 1 \,(\text{ml}) = \textbf{A} \,(\text{ml})$$

A = 8 ml
You will set the pump for 8 ml/hr.

EXAMPLE 15.3

Doctor's order reads *IV heparin 20 u/kg/hr*. Patient's weight is 64 kg. The heparin is in the standard concentration of 25 000 u/250 ml NS. This gives a concentration of 100 u/ml.

Calculate the amount of drug/hour. Multiply the dose by the patient's weight.
20 u × 64 = 1 280 u/hr
The patient will get 1 280 u/hr.

Ratio and Proportion: Means = Extremes

The known ratio is the concentration or drug (u) : volume (ml) or 100 u : 1 ml.
The unknown ratio is hourly drug (u) : hourly volume (ml) or 1 280 u : A ml.

The proportion is 1 280 u : A ml = 100 u : 1 ml

$$\begin{array}{c} \downarrow\text{-means-}\downarrow \\ 1\,280 \text{ u} : A \text{ ml} = 100 : 1 \text{ ml} \\ \uparrow\text{-------extremes-------}\uparrow \end{array}$$

Means = 100 × A = 100A
Extremes = 1 280 × 1 = 1 280

Means = Extremes   100A = 1 280
A = 12.8
The pump requires you to enter a whole number, so you will run the IV at 13 ml/hr.

Ratio and Proportion: Cross Multiplication of Fractions

When using this method, the ratio is stated in the form of a fraction.

The known ratio is 100 u in 1 ml

This is written $\dfrac{100\ (u)}{1\ (ml)}$

The unknown ratio is 1 280 u in A ml

This is written $\dfrac{1\ 280\ (u)}{A\ (ml)}$

Unknown equals known, so these fractions are equal $\dfrac{1\ 280\ (u)}{A\ (ml)} = \dfrac{100\ (u)}{1\ (ml)}$

Cross multiply $\dfrac{1\ 280\ u}{A\ ml} \nwarrow \nearrow \dfrac{100\ u}{1\ ml}$

$100A = 1\ 280$ ml
$A = 12.8$

Therefore the pump will be set to run at 13 ml/hr.

Formula

$$\dfrac{\text{Dose } \mathbf{D}\text{esired (u)}}{\text{Dose on } \mathbf{H}\text{and (u)}} \times \mathbf{S}\text{tock (ml)} = \mathbf{A}\text{mount (ml) or } \dfrac{\mathbf{D}}{\mathbf{H}} \times \mathbf{S} = \mathbf{A}$$

Dose **D**esired is 1 280 u
Dose on **H**and is 100 u
Stock is 1 ml

$$\dfrac{\mathbf{D}}{\mathbf{H}} \times \mathbf{S} = \mathbf{A} \qquad\qquad \dfrac{1\ 280\ u}{100\ u} \times 1\ \text{(ml)} = \mathbf{A}\ \text{(ml)}$$

$A = 12.8$ ml
You will set the pump for 13 ml/hr.

YOU TRY IT

(The answers to these questions are found at the end of the book.)

Calculate the IV flow rate for each of following the heparin orders. All orders will use the standard IV concentration of heparin of 25 000 u/250 ml NS.

1. Doctor's order reads *heparin IV 1 200 u/hr.*

2. Doctor's order reads *heparin IV 1 000 u/hr.*

3. Doctor's order reads *heparin IV 19u/kg/hr.* Patient's weight is 88 kg.

4. Doctor's order reads *heparin IV 17 u/kg/hr.* Patient's weight is 55 kg.

5. Doctor's order reads *heparin IV 22 u/kg/hr.* Patient's weight is 73 kg.

Other uses for heparin include treatment of unstable angina, disseminated intravascular coagulation (DIC), and myocardial infarction. Heparin is also used in conjunction with thrombolytic agents and to maintain patency of hemodialysis tubing.

KEEP IT SAFE Heparin is also used to maintain patency of vascular access devices. The preparations used for this purpose are manufactured in concentrations of 10 u/ml and 100 u/ml. They are usually called heparin lock or heparin lock flush solutions. Heparin lock solution should be used only for flushing vascular access devices. Heparin lock solutions are the only heparin preparations that should be used to flush vascular access devices.

Low Molecular Weight Heparins

Low molecular weight heparins are fragments of heparin. Each molecule weighs approximately 1/3 as much as a heparin molecule. The molecules do not bind to proteins in the serum and thus behave somewhat differently from heparin. They can be given in lower doses than heparin and do not need as frequent monitoring with APTT. They are usually given subcutaneously. Calculations of drug dosages for these medications use the same method as any other parenteral medication.

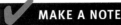

MAKE A NOTE

Most of the low molecular weight heparins are manufactured in units/ml. The exception to this is enoxaparin, Lovenox. It is manufactured in mg/ml.

Oral Anticoagulants

Coumadin (warfarin) interferes with the synthesis of Vitamin K dependent clotting factors. It acts primarily on the extrinsic and common clotting pathways. It begins to act within 24 hours of administration, but the duration of action varies from 3 to 5 days. Because of this potentially cumulative effect, it is important that this drug be monitored closely. The effect of Coumadin on the clotting mechanism is evaluated by INR. At the beginning of therapy, Coumadin orders may be written on a daily basis, after the physician has determined the daily INR.

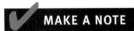

MAKE A NOTE

Many institutions have additional policies regarding the administration of anticoagulants.

They may require that anticoagulant dosages be checked by two nurses before the drug is administered. This may apply to all anticoagulants, to subcutaneous administration, or just to IV administration. Other agency policies concern the frequency of monitoring APTT and/or INR when anticoagulants are ordered. It is important to know the policies of the agency in which you are administering medications.

KEEP IT SAFE Anticoagulant therapy can be dangerous. Patients are at greater risk for bruising, bleeding, and occasionally haemorrhaging. There are a number of assessments that should be carried out frequently for patients on anticoagulant therapy, interventions to maintain safety, and patient teaching for those who are to undergo anticoagulant therapy in the community. Regular monitoring of INR and/or APTT should be carried out. INR is used to evaluate Coumadin/warfarin therapy. APTT is used to evaluate heparin therapy. The nurse should ensure that the appropriate blood test is carried out regularly.

The patient on anticoagulant therapy should be assessed for the following signs of bleeding:

- Visible bruising or petechiae
- Prolonged oozing of blood from the oral cavity, minor injuries and the insertion points of any invasive procedure
- Presence of blood in sputum, urine, and stool
- Epistaxis
- Headache, chest, abdominal, or pelvic pain that is not associated with preexisting pathology
- Prolonged or excessive menstruation

Nursing interventions for patients on anticoagulant therapy include the following:

- Use a soft toothbrush for oral care.
- Use an electric razor for shaving if INR or APPT is very high.
- Avoid injections and other invasive procedures to decrease potential for bleeding.
- Avoid mechanical trauma, e.g., pulling patient up in bed.
- Administer stool softeners as ordered to decrease straining.
- Provide high fibre foods and increased fluids to decrease constipation.
- Avoid rectal thermometers, rectal tubes, and enemas to avoid trauma to mucous membrane.
- Treat nausea, vomiting, and diarrhea aggressively to decrease GI bleeding.
- Control cough to decrease hemoptysis and orbital ecchymosis.

Health teaching for the patient in the community includes the following:

- Monitor for the above signs of bleeding and report them to the physician immediately.
- Avoid potential injury by following the above interventions.
- Many medications interact with anticoagulants to increase or decrease their effectiveness. Patients should not change their medications or take over-the-counter medications without medical supervision.
- Avoid Vitamin K rich foods such as cabbage, broccoli, asparagus, fish, liver, etc., as this will decrease the effectiveness of oral anticoagulants.
- Carry medical identification that indicates the anticoagulant use and the name and phone number of the appropriate physician.

Answers to these questions are found at the end of the book.

CASE STUDY

Elizabeth Komarovsky is a 38-year-old woman who has been admitted with a pulmonary embolus. She weighs 54 kg. Her heparin orders are as follows:

Heparin IV at 90 u/kg/hr until APPT is 2 times control, then
Heparin IV at 20 u/kg/hr to maintain target APPT.

Heparin is supplied premixed with 25 000 u of heparin in 250 ml of normal saline.

1. At what rate will you run the IV on admission?

2. At what rate will you run the IV when the target APPT is reached?

Mrs. Komarovsky's physician is monitoring her APPT twice daily. Her APPT starts to rise so he changes the order to Heparin IV at 17 u/kg/hr.

3. At what rate will you run the IV?

Three days later, the physician decides to change her heparin to subcutaneous injection. The order now reads Heparin 9 000 u sc BID. The heparin is in an ampoule labelled **Heparin 10 000 u/ml.**

4.   How much heparin will you draw up?

After a week of heparin therapy, the physician decides to change to Coumadin. The order reads Coumadin 3 mg today. You look in the medication cupboard and find that there are bottles of **Coumadin 1 mg tablets, Coumadin 2 mg tablets,** *and* **Coumadin 5 mg tablets** *available.*

5.   What combination of tablets will you pour for Mrs. Komarovsky?

OBJECTIVES

The student will:

- **calculate dosages ordered in dose/kg**

- **calculate body surface area (BSA)**

- **calculate dosages ordered in dose/m^2**

- **confirm that doctors' orders fall within the safe dosage range for children**

- **calculate appropriate fluid intake for children**

KEY TERMS

Nomogram: a chart with three variables that are represented graphically. The variables are placed in relation to each other so that connecting two known variables with a straight line gives the value of the third unknown variable.

Body surface area nomogram: a nomogram in which the known variables are height and weight. Connecting the two with a straight line gives the body surface area in metres squared.

Administration of medications to children is similar to administration to adults, in that many of the same techniques and calculations are used. There are some critical differences, however. Dosages are much smaller and the need for accuracy is much greater. Some of the techniques of administration also must be modified when the patient is a child.

We take it for granted that children do not require as large a dose of medication as an adult to achieve the same purpose. Dosages cannot be based on age, however, because of the variability in size between children of the same age. A 12-month-old girl who is 68 cm long and weighs 8 kg and a 12-month-old girl who is 78 cm long and weighs 11.6 kg are both considered to be within the norms for that age.

Two methods have been developed to identify the appropriate dosage of medications for children. These are dose/kg that is based on body weight and dose/m^2 that is based on body surface area.

MAKE A NOTE ✓

The weight and height of a child are frequently used as part of medication calculations. It is helpful to have this information readily available. Depending on the organization of the unit and the medication system, keep a note of the weight and height at each child's bedside or on each MAR.

Medications Ordered in Dose/Kilogram

The simplest way to calculate dosages for children is dosage/kg. Medications may be ordered as mg/kg or mcg/kg. In order to calculate the amount of drug, multiply the dose times the body weight in kg.

EXAMPLE 16.1

The doctor's order reads *Lanoxin (digoxin) 3.5 µg/kg po bid*. The child weighs 25 kg. The label on the bottle of medication reads **Lanoxin 50 µg/ml.**

Dose of drug (µg/kg) × weight (kg) = µg of drug

3.5 µg/kg × 25 kg = 87.5 µg of Lanoxin.

To calculate the amount of Lanoxin to administer, the same methods are used as for any liquid medication.

Ratio and Proportion: Means = Extremes

The known ratio is 50 µg : 1 ml
The unknown ratio is 87.5 µg : A ml

$$\begin{array}{c}\downarrow\text{-means-}\downarrow\\87.5 : A \quad = \quad 50 : 1\\\uparrow\text{----extremes----}\uparrow\end{array}$$

Means = Extremes
50A = 87.5
A = 1.75 ml

Ratio and Proportion: Cross Multiplication of Fractions

Known ratio is 50 μg in 1 ml: $\dfrac{50}{1}$

Unknown ratio is 87.5 μg in A ml: $\dfrac{87.5}{A}$

$\dfrac{87.\mu5 \text{ g}}{A \text{ ml}} \quad \dfrac{50 \text{ } \mu g}{1 \text{ ml}}$

50A = 87.5
A = 1.75 ml

Formula

$$\frac{\text{Dose } \mathbf{D}\text{esired } (\mu g)}{\text{Dose on } \mathbf{H}\text{and } (\mu g)} \times \mathbf{S}\text{tock (pills)} = \mathbf{A}\text{mount}$$

$$\text{or} \quad \frac{\mathbf{D}}{\mathbf{H}} \times \mathbf{S} = \mathbf{A}$$

Dose **D**esired is 87.5 μg
Dose on **H**and is 50 μg
Stock is 1 ml

$$\frac{87.5 \text{ } \mu g}{50 \text{ } \mu g} \times 1 \text{ ml} = \mathbf{A}$$

A = 1.75 ml

KEEP IT SAFE Because paediatric drugs are ordered in very small quantities, the unit of measurement is frequently micrograms, mcg or μg. The container of the drug you are using may be labelled in either micrograms or milligrams. Always check very carefully to ensure that you are always working in the same units. Convert all measurements to the same units before calculating the amount of drug to give. In the above example, digoxin elixir may be labelled 50 μg/ml or 0.05 mg/ml. It would be easy to make an error if the order were in micrograms and the label on the package in milligrams.

YOU TRY IT

(The answers to these questions are found at the end of the book.)

MEDICATIONS ORDERED IN DOSE/KG

1. Helena is a 6-month-old girl who weighs 5 kg. The doctor's order reads *gentamycin 1 mg/kg IV q12h*. The label on the vial reads **gentamycin 10 mg/ml**. How much gentamycin should you draw up?

2. Ramon is a 17-month-old boy who weighs 6.3 kg. The doctor's order reads *ondansetron 0.1 mg/kg IV q8h PRN for nausea and vomiting*. The label on the vial reads **ondansetron 2 mg/ml.** How much ondansetron should you draw up?

3. Natasha is a 3-year-old girl who weighs 14.7 kg. The doctor's order reads *Cefizox (ceftizoxime) 50 mg/kg IV Q8H*. The label on the vial reads **Cefizox 1 gram.** The dilution instructions state that you should add 3 ml of normal saline to get a concentration of 270 mg/ml. How much Cefizox should you draw up?

4. MacKenzie is a 6-year-old girl who weighs 21.4 kg. The doctor's order reads *Ceclor (cefaclor) 10 mg/kg po q8h*. The label on the bottle reads **Ceclor 375 mg/5 ml.** How much Ceclor should you administer?

5. Armand is a 10-year-old boy who weighs 35 kg. The doctor's order reads *Flagyl (metronidazole) 10 mg/kg IV*. Flagyl comes premixed in a 100-ml bag with a strength of 500 mg/100 ml. How much of the Flagyl will you administer?

Calculation of Body Surface Area (BSA)

Dosage based on body surface area is considered to be the best method of identifying the most appropriate amount of some medications for children. BSA is measured in square metres (m^2). To calculate body surface area (BSA), you can use either a body surface nomogram or a formula.

BSA is usually calculated using a body surface nomogram (Figure 16-1).

To do this, draw a straight line from the patient's height in cm on the left side of the chart to the patient's weight in kg on the right side of the chart. The point at which this line intersects the middle scale is the body surface area in m^2.

If a body surface nomogram is not available, the following formula can be used.

$$BSA\ (m^2)\ =\ \sqrt{\frac{Weight\ (kg) \times Height\ (cm)}{3\ 600}}$$

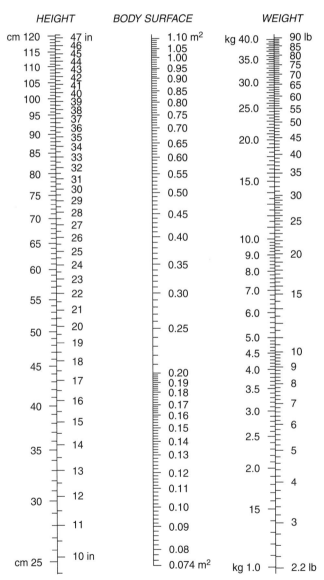

FIGURE 16-1 Pediatric body surface area nomogram. (From DuBois, D., & Dubois, F. [1916]. A formula to estimate the approximate surface area if height and weight be known. *Archives of Internal Medicine, 17,* 863–871.

EXAMPLE 16.2

John is a 9-year-old boy who is 135 cm tall and weighs 30 kg.

$$\text{BSA (m}^2) = \sqrt{\frac{\text{Weight (kg)} \times \text{Height (cm)}}{3\,600}}$$

$$= \sqrt{\frac{30 \times 135}{3\,600}}$$

$$= \sqrt{1.125}$$

$$= 1.06 \text{ m}^2$$

YOU TRY IT

(The answers to these questions are found at the end of the book.)

CALCULATION OF BODY SURFACE AREA

1. A 22-month-old girl is 82 cm tall and weighs 13 kg.

2. A 2-month-old boy is 57 cm long and weighs 4.6 kg.

3. A 5-year-old girl is 103 cm tall and weighs 16 kg.

4. A 10-year-old boy is 144 cm tall and weighs 42 kg.

5. A 15-year-old boy is 180 cm tall and weighs 75 kg.

Medications Ordered in Dose/m²

To calculate the amount of drug to give when the order is written as amount/m², multiply the dose of drug times the BSA.

Bobby is an 8-year-old boy with acute lymphocytic leukemia. He is 127 cm tall and weighs 22 kg. The doctor's order reads *methotrexate 20 mg/m² IM Q 10 days*. The label on the vial reads **methotrexate 50 mg/2 ml.**

Calculation of BSA

$$\text{BSA (m}^2) = \sqrt{\frac{\text{Weight (kg)} \times \text{Height (cm)}}{3\,600}}$$

$$\text{BSA (m}^2) = \sqrt{\frac{22 \text{ kg} \times 127 \text{ cm}}{3\,600}}$$

$$= \sqrt{0.78}$$

$$= 0.88 \text{ m}^2$$

Calculation of Dose of Drug

Amount of drug × BSA = Amount of drug in each dose

Dose of drug mg/m² × BSA (m²) = mg of drug

20 mg/m² × 0.88 m² = 17.6 mg of methotrexate

Calculation of Amount of Drug to Give

To calculate the amount of methotrexate to administer, the same methods are used as for any liquid medication.

Ratio and Proportion: Means = Extremes

The known ratio is 50 mg : 2 ml
The unknown ratio is 17.6 mg : A ml

$$\downarrow\text{-means-}\downarrow$$
$$17.6 : A \ = \ 50 : 2$$
$$\uparrow\text{---extremes----}\uparrow$$

Means = Extremes
50A = 35.2
A = 0.7 ml

Ratio and Proportion: Cross Multiplication of Fractions

Known ratio is 50 mg in 2 ml, or $\dfrac{50}{2}$

Unknown ratio is 17.6 mg in A ml, or $\dfrac{17.6}{A}$

$$\frac{17.6 \text{ mg}}{A \text{ ml}} \begin{smallmatrix}\nwarrow & \nearrow \\ \swarrow & \searrow\end{smallmatrix} \frac{50 \text{ mg}}{2 \text{ ml}}$$

50A = 35.2
A = 0.7 ml

Formula

$$\frac{\text{Dose \textbf{D}esired (mg)}}{\text{Dose on \textbf{H}and (mg)}} \times \textbf{S}\text{tock (pills)} = \textbf{A}\text{mount}$$

$$\text{or} \ \ \frac{\textbf{D}}{\textbf{H}} \times \textbf{S} = \textbf{A}$$

Dose **D**esired is 17.6 mg
Dose on **H**and is 50 mg
Stock is 2 ml

$$\frac{17.6 \text{ mg}}{50 \text{ mg}} \times 2 \text{ ml} = \textbf{A}$$

A = 0.7 ml

YOU TRY IT

(The answers to these questions are found at the end of the book.)

MEDICATIONS ORDERED IN DOSE/m²

1. Brian is 16-year-old boy with a diagnosis of Hodgkin's disease. He is 158 cm tall and weighs 43 kg. The doctor's order reads *Blenoxane (bleomycin) 15 u/m² IV twice weekly*. The label on the vial reads **Blenoxane 15 u.** The directions on the vial state that the drug should be reconstituted with 10 ml of normal saline. How much Blenoxane will your draw up?

2. Susan is a 3-year-old girl with a diagnosis of acute lymphocytic leukemia. She is 93 cm tall and weighs 12 kg. The doctor's order reads *Myleran (busulfan) 1.8 mg/m² po daily*. The label on the bottle of tablets reads **Myleran 2 mg tablets**. The package material states that the tablets may be cut in half. How many tablets of Myleran will you administer?

3. Sean is a 2-year-old boy with a diagnosis of Letterer-Siwe disease. He is 88 cm tall and weighs 13.2 kg. His doctor's orders read *vinblastine IV once weekly according to the following schedule for 5 weeks*.

June 7	*2.5 mg/m²*
June 14	*3.75 mg/m²*
June 21	*5 mg/m²*
June 28	*6.25 mg/m²*
July 5	*7.5 mg/m²*

The label on the vial reads **vinblastine 1 mg/ml**. How much vinblastine will you draw up on each date?

Confirmation of Safe Dosage Range for Children

Children do not tolerate excess or insufficient dosages of medication as well as adults. Many manufacturers identify a safe maximum dosage or a safe dosage range for children in the literature about the drug. This information is usually available in nursing drug guides and the CPS. When you get an order for a drug for a child, it is prudent to check the literature for paediatric dosage ranges and ensure that the ordered dosage falls within that range. If it does not, you should check with the doctor before administering the drug. The doctor may well have a reason for ordering a larger or smaller dosage, but it is important that you know why the dose is outside the usual safe range before administering it.

Calculation of Safe Maximum Dosage

For some drugs, the maximum amount of drug that should be given in 24 hours is identified. You must compare the amount of drug that is ordered in a 24-hour period to the amount that it is safe to give in a 24-hour period.

EXAMPLE 16.3

The doctor's order reads *Rocephin (ceftriaxone) 30 mg/kg IV Q12H*. The patient is a 7-year-old girl who weighs 25 kg. Your drug book tells you that the maximum daily dose is 2 g/day.

Calculate the Dose of the Medication (if necessary)

$$\text{Dose of drug mg/kg} \times \text{weight (kg)} = \text{mg of drug}$$

$$30 \text{ mg/kg} \times 25 \text{ kg} = 750 \text{ mg of Rocephin}$$

Calculate the Number of Doses of Drug in 24 Hours

$$\frac{24 \text{ hours}}{\text{Frequency (hours)}} = \text{Number of doses of drug}$$

$$\frac{24 \text{ hours}}{12 \text{ hours}} = 2$$

Calculate the Total Dose of Drug to Be Given in 24 Hours

$$\text{Single dose of drug} \times \text{Number of doses in 24 hours} = \text{Total dose of drug}$$

$$750 \text{ mg} \times 2 = 1\,500 \text{ mg}$$

Compare the Total Dose of the Drug to Be Given to the Maximum Safe Dose

1 500 mg = 1.5 g
Maximum safe dose is 2 g

1.5 g is less than 2 g, so the dose is safe to give.
If the drug is ordered in the same units as the maximum safe dose, start with step 2.

Calculation of Safe Dosage Range

For some drugs, a safe dosage range is identified. You must compare the dose ordered to both the minimum and the maximum safe dosages.

EXAMPLE 16.4

The doctor's order reads *Zinacef 100 mg IV Q12H*. The patient is a 4-day-old boy who weighs 3 kg. The safe dosage range for neonates is 20–100 mg/kg/day in 2 divided doses.

Calculate the Safe Minimum Daily Dose

$$\text{Safe minimum dose of drug (mg/kg)} \times \text{Weight (kg)} = \text{mg of drug}$$

$$20 \text{ mg/kg} \times 3 \text{ kg} = 60 \text{ mg}$$

Calculate the Safe Maximum Daily Dose

$$\text{Safe maximum dose of drug (mg/kg)} \times \text{weight (kg)} = \text{mg of drug}$$

$$100 \text{ mg/kg} \times 3 \text{ kg} = 300 \text{ mg}$$

Calculate the Number of Doses to Be Given in 24 Hours

$$\frac{24 \text{ hours}}{\text{Frequency (hours)}} = \text{Number of doses of drug}$$

$$\frac{24 \text{ hours}}{12 \text{ hours}} = 2$$

Calculate the Total Dose of Drug to Be Given in 24 Hours

$$\text{Single dose of drug} \times \text{Number of doses in 24 hours} = \text{Total dose of drug}$$

$$100 \text{ mg} \times 2 = 200 \text{ mg}$$

Compare the Total Dose of the Drug to Be Given to the Minimum and Maximum Safe Doses

Ensure that the same units are being used.
Minimum safe dose is 60 mg
Maximum safe dose is 300 mg
Total amount ordered is 200 mg
This amount falls between the minimum and maximum safe doses, so it is safe to give.

YOU TRY IT

(The answers to these questions are found at the end of the book.)

CALCULATION OF SAFE DOSAGE RANGE

1. Henry is 3 years old and has been admitted with croup. The doctor's order reads *acetaminophen suppository 80 mg pr Q4H PRN*. The maximum dose in 24 hours is 720 mg. If the medication is given as often as possible, will the maximum dose be exceeded?

2. Elena is a 10-year-old girl who weighs 27.5 kg. The doctor's order reads *Pepcid (famotidine) 0.5 mg/kg IV Q8H*. The maximum daily dose is 40 mg/day. Is this dose within the safe range?

3. Randi is a 5-year-old girl who weighs 18.5 kg. The doctor's order reads *Keflex (cephalexin) suspension 250 mg po qid*. The safe dosage range for this drug is 25–100 mg/kg/day. Is this dose within the safe range?

4. Jared is a 7-year-old boy who weighs 22 kg. The doctor's order reads *phenobarbital 40 mg IV QHS*. The safe dosage range for this drug is 1–3 mg/kg/day. Is this dose within the safe range?

5. Maria is a 5-year-old girl who weighs 17 kg. The doctor's order reads *penicillin 150 000 u IV Q4H*. The safe dosage range for this drug is 25 000–300 000 u/kg/day. Is this dose within the safe range?

KEEP IT SAFE Children's doses of medication are frequently very small compared to adult doses. It can be difficult to measure them accurately using the equipment intended to measure adult medications. Always choose a measuring device that is appropriate for the size of the dose.

Graduated droppers that hold 1 ml and are marked in fractions of a millilitre are most appropriate for oral doses of less than 1 ml of liquid. Graduated medication spoons that hold 5 ml and are marked in fractions of a millilitre are most appropriate for doses between 1 and 5 ml of liquid. A 1-ml, 3-ml, or 5-ml syringe can also be used to accurately measure oral liquid medications for children. A tuberculin syringe is the most appropriate syringe for IM or SC doses of less than 1 ml.

Calculation of Fluid Requirements for Children

Just as children have less tolerance for variations in drug dosage, they also have less tolerance for variations in fluid intake. The following formula is used to calculate the appropriate fluid intake for a normally hydrated child. (A dehydrated child will need more fluids, an overhydrated one less.)

Fluid Calculation Formula

100 ml/kg/day for each kg up to 10 kg
plus
50 ml/kg/day for each additional kg up to 20 kg
plus
20 ml/kg/day for each additional kg

EXAMPLE 16.5

Carlos is an 11-year-old boy who weighs 31 kg.

100 ml/kg/day for each kg up to 10 kg = 100 ml/kg × 10 kg = 1 000 ml
plus
50 ml/kg/day for each additional kg up to 20 kg = 50 ml/kg × 10 kg = 500 ml
plus
20 ml/kg/day for each additional kg = 20 ml/kg × 11 kg = 220 ml

Total fluids 1 720 ml/day

YOU TRY IT

(The answers to these questions are found at the end of the book.)

CALCULATION OF FLUID REQUIREMENTS

Identify the appropriate amount of fluids/day for the following children.

1. Jenny, who weighs 3 kg

2. Nahid, who weighs 6 kg

3. Arkady, who weighs 12 kg

4. Madeline, who weighs 18 kg

5. Dagmar, who weighs 24 kg

KEEP IT SAFE IV therapy poses a greater risk to children than to adults because of a child's lower tolerance for excess fluids. Volume control devices should always be used when administering IV fluids and medications. If a pump is not available, an IV soluset should be used. Fill the soluset with a maximum of 2 hours' worth of IV fluid and refill as necessary.

Answers to these questions are found at the end of the book.

DRUG AND SAFE DOSE CALCULATIONS

1. Jenna weighs 13 kg. The doctor's order reads *Apo-Cloxi (cloxacillin) 20 mg/kg po q6h*. Maximum safe dose is 4 g/day. The label on the bottle reads **Apo-Cloxi Suspension 125 mg/5ml.** How many mg of Apo-Cloxi will you give? How much Apo-Cloxi will you pour? How will you measure it? Is this within the safe dosage range?

2. Andrew weighs 22 kg. The doctor's order reads *rifampin 300 mg po daily*. The label on the bottle reads **rifampin 150 mg capsules.** The safe dosage range is 10–20 mg/kg/day. How many capsules will you administer? Is this dose within the safe range?

3. Marcel weighs 38 kg and is 140 cm tall. The doctor's order reads *Amicar (aminocaproic acid) 5 g IV, followed by 1 g q1h until bleeding is controlled*. The label on the vial reads **Amicar 250 mg/ml.** The maximum safe dose is 18 g/m^2/24 hours. How much Amicar will you draw up for the first dose? How much will you draw up for each subsequent dose? If the bleeding continues for 24 hours, will the maximum safe dosage range be exceeded?

4. Alice weighs 15 kg. The doctor's order reads *Septra (trimethoprim/sulfamethoxazole) 5 ml IV q6h*. The safe dosage range for Septra is 0.31–0.63 ml/kg. Is this dose within the safe range?

5. Thea weighs 9 kg. The doctor's order reads *penicillin G 125 000 u IV q4h*. The label on the vial reads **penicillin G 1 000 000 u.** It is to be reconstituted with 3 ml of sterile water. How much penicillin will you draw up? The safe dosage range for penicillin G is 25 000–300 000 u/kg in 24 hours. Is this dose within the safe range?

FLUID INTAKE CALCULATIONS

Calculate the appropriate fluid intake for the following children.

1. Helena, who weighs 4.7 kg

2. Anneka, who weighs 7.7 kg

3. Robby, who weighs 11.4 kg

4. Jamie, who weighs 16.2 kg

5. Kayla, who weighs 18.4 kg

6. Shawna, who weighs 22.5 kg

7. Lili, who weighs 24 kg

8. Pierre, who weighs 25.8 kg

9. Gurmant, who weighs 28 kg

10. Elizabeth, who weighs 35 kg

CASE STUDY

Andrew is a 5-year-old boy who is being treated for exacerbation of acute lymphocytic leukemia. He is 110 cm tall and weighs 16 kg. His doctor's orders are as follows:

AGH
Anywhere General Hospital

0239705
Zaleski, Andrew
44 Coleman St.
Apt 16
Anywhere, Ontario

Doctor's Orders

Date	Orders
Feb 2/05	Days 1–7 inclusive
	Cytostar 100 mg/m² IV od
	Days 1–3 inclusive
	Adriamycin 30 mg/m² IV od
	Days 1–5 inclusive
	Solu–cortef 40 mg/m² IV bid
	Days 1 and 5
	vincristine 1.5 mg/m² od
	A.K. Gryffe MD

The labels on the medication containers read as follows:

Cytostar (cytarabine) 100 mg vial. Dilute with 5 ml of NS for a concentration of 20 mg/ml

Adriamycin (doxyrubacin) 50 mg/25 ml

Solu-cortef (hydrocortisone) Act-O-Vial. When mixed, each vial contains 100 mg/2 ml vincristine 1 mg/ml in each 2-ml vial.

Identify which drugs you will give on each day of this 7-day course of chemotherapy. Identify the dose of the drug and the amount of solution you will draw up.

Andrew must be well hydrated during this course of chemotherapy. How much fluid should he have each day?

Administration of Blood and Blood Products

OBJECTIVES

The student will:

■ describe the system used in Canada for collection and administration of blood and blood products

■ describe the potential acute complications associated with administration of blood and blood products and the interventions used to decrease those complications

■ describe, know the procedure for administration, and carry out the appropriate calculations for the following blood products:
  • packed red blood cells
  • fresh frozen plasma
  • platelets
  • albumin
  • cryoprecipitate
  • factor concentrates

KEY TERMS

Erythrocytes or red blood cells: cells containing hemoglobin which circulate in the vascular system, transporting oxygen and carbon dioxide.

Leukocytes or white blood cells: a group of circulating cells that play a major role in inflammation and immune response.

Thrombocytes or platelets: circulating cell fragments that play a major role in blood clotting.

ABO group: classification of blood according to the antigens on the surface of red cells and the corresponding antibody. There are two antigens, A and B. Blood cells may have either A or B, both A and B, or no antigens. Those who have A antigens on the red cells, have anti-B antibodies. Those with B have anti-A, and so on. The mixing of red cells with blood containing the antibody for those cells will cause agglutination, or clumping together, of the red cells. Subsequent breakdown of the agglutinated red cells causes severe illness or death.

Rh group: eighty-five percent of people have the Rh antigen on the surface of their red cells. These people are known as Rh positive. Fifteen percent of people have no Rh antigen and are Rh negative. When a person with Rh negative blood is exposed to Rh positive blood, the body starts to make anti-Rh antibodies. Not enough antibodies are made during the first exposure to cause problems, but subsequent exposure will cause agglutination of the transfused Rh positive cells.

Transfusion: the infusion of blood or a blood product into the vascular system.

Hematocrit: the percentage of blood that is composed of cells. The normal hematocrit is 42%–50% for men and 40%–48% for women.

Apheresis: a process in which the blood that is removed from the donor is immediately passed through a machine that removes a selected blood component. The remainder of the blood is then returned to the donor.

Plasmapheresis: apheresis in which plasma is collected from a donor.

Plateletpheresis: apheresis in which platelets are collected from a donor.

Osmolality: the osmotic pressure of a solution. Osmotic pressure causes the movement of a solvent (water), across a semipermeable membrane, from an area of low concentration of solute (particles) to an area of high concentration of solute.

Clotting factors: proteins that circulate in the bloodstream in an inactive state. When the clotting mechanism is triggered, the clotting factors become active in a sequential fashion that leads to the development of a fibrin clot.

Blood and blood products are used to replace blood loss or to provide patients with elements of blood that they are not able to produce themselves. Blood cannot be manufactured; it must be obtained from a donor and then administered to the patient.

Canadian Blood Collection and Distribution System

The collection, storage, and distribution of blood and blood products in Canada is carried out by Canadian Blood Services (CBS). CBS is a not-for-profit organization whose sole mission is to manage the blood and blood product supply for Canadians.

Blood is collected from volunteer donors at clinics that are run by CBS. The blood is tested for a variety of infectious diseases and for ABO and Rh group. Each unit of blood is processed and separated into a variety of component parts. Some blood components are collected through a process called *apheresis*. This is a process in which the blood that is removed from the donor is immediately passed through a machine that removes a selected blood component. The remainder of the blood is then returned to the donor.

Because blood is a form of human tissue, it is fragile and perishable and must be handled carefully in order for it to be safe and effective. When it is needed, it is shipped to the appropriate setting where it is administered to those who need it. There is no charge to the patient.

Potential Acute Complications Associated with Blood and Blood Products

Haemolytic Reaction

A haemolytic reaction is caused when the ABO group of the donor blood is different from the ABO group of the recipient, or when there is an Rh incompatibility. When the blood is infused into the patient, the recipient antibodies are incompatible with transfused red cells. This causes the red cells to agglutinate or clump together. The signs and symptoms include the rapid onset of increased temperature, increased blood pressure, dyspnea, and back pain.

Haemolytic reactions are prevented by carrying out appropriate diagnostic testing. The donated blood is typed for ABO and Rh group. When a specific unit of blood is designated for a specific patient, the patient is typed for ABO and Rh group, then the cells of the donor blood are mixed with the serum of the recipient to see whether agglutination occurs. This test is called *cross-matching*. Once the lab has determined that this unit of blood is appropriate for this specific patient, two nurses must check the label on the blood and the patient arm band to ensure that the correct patient receives the blood.

Haemolytic reaction is fortunately very rare. Since it is potentially fatal, appropriate precautions must always be taken to prevent it.

Febrile Reaction

Febrile reactions are caused by recipient sensitivity to antigens on white cells or platelets in donor blood. The incidence increases with the number of transfusions. The signs and symptoms include tachycardia, peripheral vasodilation, shaking, and increased temperature.

In order to decrease the incidence of febrile reactions, CBS removes most of the leukocytes from the units of packed red cells.

Bacterial Contamination

While bacterial contamination is quite rare, it is possible for blood to become contaminated at some point during the collection, processing, and distribution process. The signs and symptoms are those of acute systemic infection and may proceed to septic shock.

Warm temperature increases bacterial growth, so blood is stored at less than 6°C. Specific time limits for administration have been identified for various blood products (see below). These time limits must be observed, even though it may be inconvenient to do so.

Allergic Reaction

Allergic reactions occur when the recipient has an immune response to foreign serum protein or when there is a transfer of an antigen or reaginic antibody from donor to recipient. Signs and symptoms of allergic reaction to blood products are the same as those for any allergic reaction: urticaria, bronchospasm, dyspnea, and circulatory collapse.

Patients with a history of allergies are frequently given an antihistamine or (in more severe cases) a glucocorticoid before the blood product is administered.

Fluid Volume Excess

Patients who are getting multiple transfusions for anemia or other problems not related to volume loss may end up with fluid volume excess. The signs and symptoms include edema, dyspnea, orthopnea, and crackles on auscultation.

Diuretics may be administered before or between transfusions to decrease the chance of fluid volume excess.

Ventricular Fibrillation

Blood and most blood products are stored at less than 6°C. When they are administered rapidly, the cold may cause ventricular fibrillation. Those most at risk are seniors and those with pre-existing cardiac arrhythmias.

Ventricular fibrillation can be prevented by administering the blood at a slower rate. Blood products can be warmed using a heater which warms the blood as it passes through the tubing. Never warm blood in a microwave or in a bowl of warm water. It is also inappropriate to warm blood by letting it sit at room temperature for a period of time.

Other Complications

The above complications are those most likely to occur at the time of transfusion. In addition, there are a number of longer-term complications that can occur:

- Hemosiderosis is an excess accumulation of iron that occurs in patients with haemolytic anemia who require multiple transfusions.
- Transfusion-related lung injury is a form of acute respiratory distress syndrome which occurs as a result of antibodies in the donor plasma.
- Graft-versus-host disease occurs when the donor leukocytes attack the host tissues. It usually occurs in severely immunocompromised patients.
- There are a number of infectious diseases that may be transmitted through blood and blood products. These include HIV, hepatitis B and C, syphilis, West Nile virus, and human T-cell lymphotropic virus (HTLV). Donors must fill out a health and lifestyle questionnaire before donating blood. CBS then tests the blood for these diseases before the blood is processed.

For the signs and symptoms and treatment of the above complications, consult a medical-surgical nursing textbook.

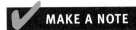

MAKE A NOTE

The procedures suggested here are general guidelines. Always check the agency pro-cedure manual for the specific procedure associated with administration of blood and blood products.

Blood Products

Whole Blood

Whole blood contains red blood cells, plasma, and citrate, an anticoagulation preser-vative. It is used to restore whole blood losses such as occur during haemorrhage because it replaces both volume and oxygen-carrying capacity. It has a hematocrit of 35–40% and must be ABO compatible with the recipient. Whole blood is rarely used and is not usually stocked in most institutions. The procedure for administration of whole blood is the same as for packed red cells.

Packed Red Cells

A unit of packed red cells is whole blood with most of the plasma removed. This is the product usually referred to as a *blood transfusion*. The most common form of trans-fusion therapy, it is used for people with anemia or other diseases where there is impairment of blood cell production or accelerated blood cell destruction. It provides the most O_2 carrying capacity in the smallest volume. It must be ABO compatible with the recipient. It should also be Rh compatible for Rh negative recipients.

Each unit contains approx 250–300 ml of packed cells and will raise the hemoglo-bin level by approximately 10 gm/L. The hematocrit of packed cells is approximately 75–80%. Packed cells must be used within 42 days of collection.

To administer a transfusion of packed red cells, you must first start an IV using a large-bore (18 gauge) needle. Specialized tubing called Y tubing is used for the trans-fusion. The blood is attached to one arm of the Y and normal saline is attached to the other (Figure 17-1). The tubing is primed with the normal saline and the normal saline should run at a slow rate of 30–50 ml/hr until the blood is hung. Only normal saline is used with blood products. IV solutions containing either glucose or calcium are dam-aging to the blood. Medications or TPN are never added to blood, nor should blood be administered through tubing that has been used for anything other than normal saline. Most blood products, including red cells, must be stored at 6°C or lower. In most institutions, there is a special refrigerator in the lab which is carefully tempera-ture controlled and is used only for blood products. The blood should not be taken from this refrigerator until the patient's IV line is established.

Once the IV is started, the blood is brought from the lab to the patient's bedside. Two nurses check the blood bag, the lab slips, and the patient to ensure that the blood is being given to the right patient. Packed cells should be run over a period of two to three hours. If the blood hangs for more than four hours, it should be taken down and discarded, even if it is not finished. The blood should be run slowly (40 ml/hr) for the first 15 minutes so that if the patient develops a severe reaction, he or she will not have had a lot of blood. Blood tubing usually has a drip factor of 10. You should assume that the blood bag will have approximately 300 ml in it. Calculations for drip rate are in two parts.

1. Drip rate for the first 15 minutes

$$\frac{\text{Amount of fluid (ml)} \times \text{Drip factor (gtts/ml)}}{\text{Time in hours} \times 60 \text{ minutes}} = \text{Drip rate (gtts/min)}$$

$$\frac{40 \text{ ml} \times 10}{1 \text{ hour} \times 60 \text{ minutes}} = 7 \text{ gtts/min}$$

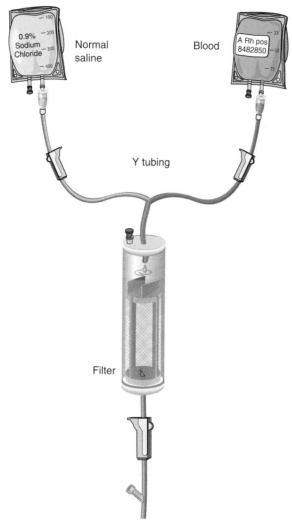

FIGURE 17-1 Y tubing.

2. Drip rate for the transfusion

$$\frac{\text{Amount of fluid (ml)} \times \text{Drip factor (gtts/ml)}}{\text{Time in hours} \times 60 \text{ minutes}} = \text{Drip rate (gtts/min)}$$

$$\frac{300 \text{ ml} \times 10}{3 \text{ hours} \times 60 \text{ minutes}} = 17 \text{ gtts/min}$$

If you are using a pump to administer the blood, set it for 40 ml/hr for the first 15 minutes and then 100 ml/hour for the remainder of the transfusion.

Because there are a number of potential complications associated with blood and blood product therapy, assessment of the patient before and during the transfusion is critically important. Nursing assessment of patients receiving blood products should include

- vital signs
  - temperature
  - pulse
  - respirations
  - blood pressure
- chest auscultation
- monitoring the patient for complaints of
  - pain
  - chills

- itching
- headache

Assessment should be carried out before the transfusion starts, 15 minutes after the beginning of the transfusion, and regularly thereafter. Check agency policy for the frequency of monitoring. If there is no agency policy, assess the patient every half-hour for the first hour and every hour thereafter.

If the patient shows a significant change between assessments, especially increased temperature accompanied by altered blood pressure and back or chest pain, stop the transfusion and call the doctor. To stop the transfusion, clamp off the blood tubing. Prime a new set of tubing with normal saline and attach the line into the port closest to the insertion site of the IV. This will maintain the IV site without introducing any more blood product into the patient.

KEEP IT SAFE Blood should always be administered through a dedicated IV line that is not used for medication administration. Medications are incompatible with blood and are never added to an IV line that is running blood.

Fresh Frozen Plasma

Plasma is the liquid portion of the blood. It contains a number of proteins, called plasma proteins, that have a wide variety of functions in the body. It is used for volume replacement in shock and severe burns. It is also used to treat liver disease, and in some types of cancer therapy. It must be ABO compatible.

Plasma may be collected during a whole blood donation. The unit of blood is centrifuged; part of it becomes a unit of packed cells and part of it becomes fresh frozen plasma. This is usually called *recovered plasma*. Most plasma, however, is collected through an apheresis process called *plasmapheresis*. This produces two to three times more plasma than a standard blood donation.

Plasma is frozen immediately after it is taken from the donor. It is stored frozen for up to a year until a specific patient requires it. It takes approximately 30 minutes to thaw and prepare a unit of plasma for administration. Once it is thawed, the transfusion should begin immediately and should not last longer than 4 hours.

A unit of fresh frozen plasma contains approximately 250 ml. The procedure for administering plasma and the associated assessments are the same as for transfusions of packed red cells.

Platelets

Platelets are cellular fragments that are an essential part of the clotting mechanism. Some patients have platelets that do not function properly; others have diseases or have undergone treatments that cause the platelets to break down too quickly. These patients may need a transfusion of platelets to maintain normal blood clotting.

Platelets are the most fragile of the blood products. They are usually collected through plateletpheresis. A unit of platelets must be used within 5 days of collection, must be continually agitated during storage, and must be stored at 20–24°C. It must be ABO compatible. Some patients who need frequent transfusions of platelets develop antibodies which can lead to anaphylaxis. Platelet transfusions for these patients must be matched by human leukocyte antigen (HLA) type as well as ABO.

Platelets are usually administered over approximately 30 minutes. The maximum time for an infusion of platelets is 4 hours. The procedure and assessment is the same for platelets as it is for packed red cells.

Albumin

Albumin is a plasma protein that maintains the osmolality of the blood and also acts as a transport mechanism to carry substances, including medications, around the body. Patients who lack sufficient albumin can develop serious shifts of fluid out of the vascular system into the interstitial and third spaces.

Albumin is removed from donor blood and concentrated for administration. It is available in two strengths: 5% and 25%. Five percent albumin comes in 50 ml and 250 ml vials, while 25% is packaged in 50 ml and 100 ml vials. It does not have to be ABO compatible.

Albumin is packaged with a vented administration set and should be administered using an infusion pump. The rate of infusion is by doctor's order.

In addition to the usual assessment of a patient receiving a transfusion, it is important to assess for rapid fluid shifts. The high osmolality of the albumin will pull fluid out of body cavities, especially the abdominal cavity, and return it to circulation.

Cryoprecipitate

Blood clotting is dependent on proteins that normally circulate in the blood in an inactive form. When the clotting mechanism is triggered by trauma or other stimuli, the inactive proteins become active in a sequential manner. If a patient is deficient in one or more of the clotting proteins (usually called *clotting factors*), the mechanism is unable to go forward and a clot is not formed. Hemophilia A and B and von Willebrand's disease are the commonest of these problems.

Cryoprecipitate is a concentrated solution of a number of clotting factors in a small amount of plasma. It is used to control bleeding in patients with clotting disorders. Cryoprecipitate is stored frozen and thawed when required. Once thawed, it should be administered immediately and should not hang for more than 4 hours. It should not be refrigerated after thawing, as this will cause the clotting factors to separate out from the plasma. ABO testing is preferable but not essential.

One unit of cryoprecipitate is 10 ml; the total number of units ordered by the physician will be pooled in one bag in the lab. Y tubing is used for cryoprecipitate. The infusion should be run rapidly over not more than 1 hour. The tubing should be flushed with normal saline after the transfusion to ensure that the patient receives all of it. The assessment of a patient receiving cryoprecipitate is the same as for patients receiving packed red cells.

Factor Concentrates

Cryoprecipitate used to be the preferred treatment for patients with clotting disorders. In recent years, however, it has become possible to isolate, store, and administer individual clotting factors. Canadian Blood Services supplies a variety of products of this type. Most of them are administered by direct IV administration over 3–5 minutes. ABO compatibility is not required. Patients with chronic disease can be taught to self-administer these products as necessary.

chapter 17

Self Test

Answers to these questions are found at the end of the book.

Match the potential complication associated with blood transfusion with the measures usually taken to prevent them.

1. Haemolytic reaction
2. Febrile reaction
3. Bacterial contamination
4. Allergic reaction
5. Fluid volume excess

A. Administration of antihistamines
B. Blood is stored at 6°C
C. Blood is typed for ABO and Rh group and each unit is cross-matched to the individual recipient
D. Administration of diuretics
E. Most of the leukocytes are removed from the units of packed cells

6. What is the only IV solution that can be administered with blood?

7. Which blood component has a lifespan of only 5 days?

8. Which blood component can cause a significant shift of fluid from the abdominal cavity into the vascular system?

9. Identify the components of the nursing assessment that should be carried out on any patient who is receiving a transfusion of blood or blood products.

10. What is the appropriate flow rate for an infusion of packed cells that is being run on a pump?

18 Parenteral Nutrition

OBJECTIVES

The student will:

- know the indications for total and partial parenteral nutrition

- describe the solutions used for parenteral nutrition

- identify the complications associated with parenteral nutrition

- describe the assessment of a patient receiving parenteral nutrition

KEY TERMS

Anorexia-cachexia syndrome: syndrome occurring in the end stage of cancer characterized by extreme weight loss and wasting.

Peripherally inserted central catheter (PICC): venous access device which is inserted into a peripheral vein and threaded through the vascular system to the right vena cava.

Centrally inserted catheter: venous access device which is tunnelled through the subcutaneous tissue of the chest, inserted into a major vein and directed into the right vena cava.

Multilumen access device: peripheral or central catheter which has more than one cavity or channel through the catheter. Each channel can be used for a separate purpose, such as administration of different medications and/or parenteral nutrition.

Azotemia: excess urea and other nitrogenous compounds in the blood.

Parenteral nutrition is the provision of nutrients via the vascular system. It is used when patients are unable to take in sufficient nutrients by mouth. This may be as a result of gastrointestinal tract dysfunction, increased metabolic demand, or a combination of both. Some of the major indications for parenteral nutrition are as follows:

- gastrointestinal fistula
- inadequate absorption due to short bowel syndrome or malabsorption syndrome
- bowel obstruction
- need for prolonged bowel rest such as pancreatitis
- severe malnutrition
- anorexia-cachexia syndrome
- multiple trauma
- major burns
- after bowel surgery

Total parenteral nutrition (TPN) is used when a patient is unable to take in or absorb any nutrient. All of the nutritional needs are met by the TPN. Partial parenteral nutrition (PPN) is used for patients who are able to take in some nutrients by the GI tract but still need supplements. The calculation of a patient's nutritional needs is carried out by a dietitian who consults with the doctor to identify the appropriate solution and the amounts to be given.

Total Parenteral Nutrition (TPN)

The basic elements of TPN are amino acids, glucose and lipids. In addition, most TPN solutions include a variety of electrolytes. The bag containing the amino acid/glucose solution is manufactured and stored in two parts. The upper part of the bag contains the glucose, the lower part the amino acids and electrolytes. To administer the solution, the clamp separating the two parts is removed and the bag is gently rotated. The solution is only stable for 24 hours, so this should not be done until shortly before administration. In some settings, this is done in the pharmacy department: in others it is carried out by the nurse immediately before administration.

The amino acid/glucose solution comes in two strengths. TPN is usually carried out with the stronger solution of 4.25% amino acid and 25% glucose. Because of the high osmolality of this solution, it must be administered through a central access device such as a peripherally inserted central catheter (PICC line) or a centrally inserted catheter. The lower concentration of 3.5% amino acid and 5% glucose can be administered centrally or peripherally.

Most frequently, TPN is supplied as two solutions: a bag containing amino acids, glucose, and electrolytes and a separate bottle containing the lipids. (There is a product where the amino acids, glucose, and lipids are all in one container, but this is used much less frequently.) The lipids are packaged in a glass bottle because they interact with the plastic used in IV bags. They also come in two strengths, 10% and 20%.

In most settings, TPN may only be administered using an IV pump. The amino acid/glucose mixture is hung as the primary line and the lipids are hung as the secondary. The two solutions run concurrently. A doctor's order for TPN should include the strength and the hourly rate of each solution.

A small number of medications may be added to the amino acid/glucose solution. These include insulin, heparin, and multivitamins. They are usually added to the bag by the pharmacy department. If the medications are to be added by the nurse, the usual calculations for correct dosage should be followed (see Chapter 9). Medications should be added to a new bag before it is hung. They should not be added to a partially used bag which is in the process of infusing as it is almost impossible to ensure that the correct concentration is achieved.

KEEP IT SAFE Most patients who require TPN or PPN are ill enough to require other medications as well. Unfortunately, very few medications are compatible with TPN solutions. As a matter of safe practice, medications should not be introduced into tubing that is being used for TPN. If a multilumen access device is being used, one port should be designated for the TPN and another for medications. They should not be interchanged.

Patients who are receiving PPN through a peripheral line should have a second IV started for medications.

In many settings, agency policy requires that the TPN order, the bag label, and the patient's arm band be checked by two nurses.

Partial Parenteral Nutrition (PPN)

The patient who is able to take in some nutrients via the GI tract, but not enough to meet all of his nutritional needs, may be treated with PPN. PPN also uses both amino acid/glucose and lipid solutions, but only those which are less concentrated. It can be administered either through a central line or a peripheral line. The high osmolality of parenteral nutrition is damaging to veins, so a peripheral line usually needs to be changed frequently.

Potential Complications of Parenteral Nutrition

There are a number of potential complications of parenteral nutrition. These problems may be mechanical ones that arise from the vascular access equipment, or metabolic issues arising from the effects of the solution on body systems. Many of the metabolic problems arise if the TPN is infused too rapidly at the beginning of therapy. It takes some time for the body to adjust to a significant change in the amount of nutrients available. For this reason, starting therapy at a slow rate and increasing it gradually will decrease the incidence of a number of the metabolic problems.

Mechanical Complications

Thrombophlebitis/Thrombosis/Embolus

High osmolality fluids tend to cause inflammation of veins, particularly at the point of access. Venous inflammation can trigger the clotting mechanism, causing a fixed or free clot. The signs and symptoms include heat, pains, swelling, and redness at the access device entry point.

Infection/Sepsis

With its high protein and high sugar content, TPN solution is an ideal growth medium for bacteria. Microorganisms can be introduced into the bag of solution or into the delivery equipment any time there is a breach in the system. Special care must be taken during bag, tubing, and dressing changes to ensure that there is no contamination of the system. Tubing should be changed every 48 hours to decrease the possibility of bacterial growth. The usual signs and symptoms of systemic infection include chills, fever, tachycardia, and malaise.

Inappropriate Central Catheter Placement

If the central catheter is not placed accurately, it can result in hemothorax, pneumothorax, or cardiac dysfunction. The placement of the central catheter should always be checked by X-ray before TPN solution or any other fluid is infused.

Metabolic Complications

Fluid Volume Disturbances

The high osmolality of the solutions acts to pull water out of the cells, leaving them dehydrated. Intravascular volume increases. Patients with cellular dehydration will show decreased skin turgor, thirst, and cognitive deficits. Urine output may increase as the kidneys excrete the excess circulating volume. Patients who require large amounts of TPN may develop a fluid volume excess from the large quantities required. In these cases you may see increased turgor and dependent or pulmonary edema.

Hyperglycemia

This is most often seen when 25% glucose is used. The body is unable to respond quickly enough to move the glucose into the cells. Insulin is frequently added to the amino acid/glucose solution to help deal with this problem.

Electrolyte Disturbances

The electrolyte composition of the TPN solution must be carefully managed to ensure that the patient does not develop an excess or deficit in a wide variety of electrolytes. These include sodium, potassium, magnesium, calcium, phosphate, and chloride.

Azotemia

A sudden increase in amino acid intake can cause excess circulating nitrogenous wastes. This is most likely to happen if there is already some compromise in renal function.

Liver Dysfunction

The liver may also have difficulty dealing with a sudden increase in nutrients. Liver dysfunction may cause an increase in liver enzymes. This is a short-term problem for most patients, but TPN can cause permanent liver damage in some patients and they may not be able to continue on long-term TPN therapy.

Assessment of Patients Receiving Total or Partial Parenteral Nutrition

Patients receiving TPN or PPN require close assessment and monitoring for potential complications. Before beginning therapy, the following blood work should be carried out: CBC, PT, INR, Na, K, Mg, Cl, Ca, Ph, BUN, serum creatinine, albumin, total protein, blood sugar, alkaline phosphatase, AST, LDH, bilirubin. These levels should be monitored frequently as long as the therapy continues.

Nursing assessment should be carried out frequently and includes the following:

- Vital signs q4h
- Daily weight
- Daily glucometer
- Chest sounds
- Strict monitoring of intake and output
- Daily inspection of the insertion site of the vascular access device

chapter

18 Self Test

Answers to these questions are found at the end of the book.

1. Which component of TPN is packaged in a glass bottle?

2. Once the amino acids and glucose have been mixed, for how long is the solution stable?

3. What strength of amino acid/glucose solution can be administered either centrally or peripherally?

4. Your patient is receiving PPN through a peripheral IV line. He appears to be developing an infection, so the doctor orders *Rocephin (ceftriaxone) 1 g IV q12h*. What steps will you take to carry out this order?

5. You will assess the access device entry point at least once per shift. What signs and symptoms will you assess for?

6. Insulin may be added to TPN solution in response to what potential problem?

7. What diagnostic testing is routinely carried out to monitor for the above problem?

8. What potential problem can occur in patients who have compromised renal function?

9. What potential problem may cause pulmonary edema?

10. What assessments are carried out to monitor for the above problem?

CHAPTER 1

MANIPULATING FRACTIONS

Change the following improper fractions to mixed numbers.

1. $\dfrac{7}{3} = 2\dfrac{1}{3}$ 2. $\dfrac{6}{4} = 1\dfrac{2}{4}$ 3. $\dfrac{23}{9} = 2\dfrac{5}{9}$ 4. $\dfrac{30}{5} = 6$ 5. $\dfrac{17}{6} = 2\dfrac{5}{6}$

Change the following mixed numbers to improper fractions

6. $2\dfrac{7}{8} = \dfrac{23}{8}$ 7. $1\dfrac{1}{4} = \dfrac{5}{4}$ 8. $6\dfrac{9}{16} = \dfrac{105}{16}$ 9. $10\dfrac{23}{25} = \dfrac{273}{25}$ 10. $3\dfrac{3}{5} = \dfrac{18}{5}$

Find the lowest common denominator for the following pairs of fractions and identify which of the fractions is larger.

11. $\dfrac{4}{7}$ and $\dfrac{6}{11}$ The lowest common denominator is **77**. $\dfrac{4}{7} = \dfrac{44}{77}, \dfrac{6}{11} = \dfrac{42}{77}$

44 is larger than 42 so $\dfrac{4}{7}$ **is larger** than $\dfrac{6}{11}$

12. $\dfrac{4}{5}$ and $\dfrac{9}{10}$ The lowest common denominator is **10**. $\dfrac{4}{5} = \dfrac{8}{10}$

9 is larger than 10 so $\dfrac{9}{10}$ **is larger** than $\dfrac{4}{5}$

13. $\dfrac{7}{9}$ and $\dfrac{3}{4}$ The lowest common denominator is **36**. $\dfrac{7}{9} = \dfrac{28}{36}, \dfrac{3}{4} = \dfrac{27}{36}$

28 is larger than 27, so $\dfrac{7}{9}$ **is larger** than $\dfrac{3}{4}$.

14. $\dfrac{5}{8}$ and $\dfrac{7}{10}$ The lowest common denominator is **40**. $\dfrac{5}{8} = \dfrac{25}{40}, \dfrac{7}{10} = \dfrac{28}{40}$

28 is larger than 25 so $\dfrac{7}{10}$ **is larger** than $\dfrac{5}{8}$.

15. $\dfrac{2}{3}$ and $\dfrac{4}{6}$ The lowest common denominator is **6**. $\dfrac{2}{3} = \dfrac{4}{6}$

The fractions are **equal.**

ADDING AND SUBTRACTING FRACTIONS

Reduce the answer to the lowest common denominator.

1. $\dfrac{3}{4} - \dfrac{2}{3} = \dfrac{9}{12} - \dfrac{8}{12} = \dfrac{1}{12}$

2. $\dfrac{4}{5} + \dfrac{6}{8} + \dfrac{7}{10} = \dfrac{32}{40} + \dfrac{30}{40} + \dfrac{28}{40} = \dfrac{90}{40} = 2\dfrac{1}{4}$

3. $3\dfrac{3}{4} + \dfrac{3}{5} + \dfrac{3}{6} = \dfrac{15}{4} + \dfrac{3}{5} + \dfrac{3}{6} = \dfrac{225}{60} + \dfrac{36}{60} + \dfrac{30}{60} = \dfrac{291}{60} = 4\dfrac{51}{60}$

4. $7\dfrac{1}{2} - 5\dfrac{3}{5} = \dfrac{15}{2} - \dfrac{28}{5} = \dfrac{75}{10} - \dfrac{56}{10} = \dfrac{19}{10} = 1\dfrac{9}{10}$

5. $6\dfrac{4}{6} + 3\dfrac{5}{9} + 7\dfrac{7}{12} = \dfrac{40}{6} + \dfrac{32}{9} + \dfrac{91}{12} = \dfrac{240}{36} + \dfrac{128}{36} + \dfrac{273}{36} = \dfrac{641}{36} = 17\dfrac{29}{36}$

MULTIPLYING FRACTIONS

Reduce the answer to the lowest common denominator.

1. $\dfrac{4}{9} \times \dfrac{7}{12} = \dfrac{28}{108} = \dfrac{7}{27}$ 2. $\dfrac{6}{10} \times \dfrac{11}{12} = \dfrac{66}{120} = \dfrac{11}{20}$ 3. $\dfrac{55}{60} \times \dfrac{92}{100} = \dfrac{5\,060}{6\,000} = \dfrac{253}{300}$

4. $\dfrac{12}{36} \times \dfrac{15}{30} = \dfrac{180}{1\,080} = \dfrac{1}{6}$ 5. $\dfrac{13}{15} \times \dfrac{17}{19} = \dfrac{221}{285}$

DIVIDING FRACTIONS

Reduce the answer to the lowest common denominator.

1. $\dfrac{4}{9} \div \dfrac{7}{12} = \dfrac{4}{9} \times \dfrac{12}{7} = \dfrac{48}{63} = \dfrac{16}{21}$ 2. $\dfrac{6}{10} \div \dfrac{11}{12} = \dfrac{6}{10} \times \dfrac{12}{11} = \dfrac{72}{110} = \dfrac{36}{55}$

3. $\dfrac{55}{60} \div \dfrac{92}{100} = \dfrac{55}{60} \times \dfrac{100}{92} = \dfrac{5\,500}{5\,520} = \dfrac{275}{276}$ 4. $\dfrac{12}{36} \div \dfrac{15}{30} = \dfrac{12}{36} \times \dfrac{30}{15} = \dfrac{360}{540} = \dfrac{2}{3}$

5. $\dfrac{13}{15} \div \dfrac{17}{19} = \dfrac{13}{15} \times \dfrac{19}{17} = \dfrac{247}{255}$

ROUNDING OFF DECIMALS

1. 17.638 round off to 2 decimal places = **17.64**

2. 4.0028 round off to 2 decimal places = **4**

3. 0.4555 round off to 3 decimal places = **0.456**

4. 3.3333333333 round off to 2 decimal places = **3.33**

5. 0.25 round off to 1 decimal place = **0.3**

ADDING AND SUBTRACTING DECIMALS

1. 51.06 + 19.44 + 21.73 = **92.23**   2. 14.75 + 12.25 = **27**

3. 22.33 + 44.33 + 66.33 = **132.99**   4. 12.575 + 75.05 + 9.4 = **97.025**

5. 30.03 + 19.02 + 12.375 = **61.425**   6. 54.09 − 22.36 = **31.73**

7. 33.33 − 30.003 = **3.327**   8. 65.011 − 12.2 = **52.811**

9. 48.67 − 39.4 = **9.27**   10. 68.77 − 54.098 = **14.672**

MULTIPLYING DECIMALS

Round off the answer to two decimal places.

1. $16.44 \times 14.3 = \mathbf{235.09}$ 2. $5.75 \times 15.5 = \mathbf{89.13}$ 3. $42.77 \times 33.33 = \mathbf{1\ 425.52}$

4. $6.66 \times 12.5 = \mathbf{83.25}$ 5. $20.02 \times 4.11 = \mathbf{82.28}$

DIVIDING DECIMALS

Round off the answer to two decimal places.

1. $56.45 \div 2.4 = \mathbf{23.52}$ 2. $133.3 \div 15.75 = \mathbf{8.46}$ 3. $675 \div 0.125 = \mathbf{5\ 400}$

4. $336.6 \div 13.2 = \mathbf{25.5}$ 5. $455.8 \div 22.25 = \mathbf{20.49}$

CONVERTING DECIMALS TO FRACTIONS

Convert the following decimals to fractions. Reduce the fractions to the lowest common denominator.

1. $3.33 = 3\frac{33}{100}$ 2. $6.66 = 6\frac{66}{100} = 6\frac{33}{50}$ 3. $0.458 = \frac{458}{1\ 000} = \frac{229}{500}$

4. $0.083 = \frac{83}{1\ 000}$ 5. $0.625 = \frac{625}{1\ 000} = \frac{5}{8}$

CONVERTING FRACTIONS TO DECIMALS

Convert the following fractions to decimals. State the answer to two decimal places.

1. $\frac{2}{3} = \mathbf{0.67}$ 2. $\frac{6}{8} = \mathbf{0.75}$ 3. $\frac{25}{45} = \mathbf{0.56}$ 4. $\frac{93}{125} = \mathbf{0.74}$ 5. $\frac{468}{500} = \mathbf{0.94}$

CONVERTING BETWEEN DECIMALS TO PERCENT

Convert the following decimals to percent:

1. $0.13 = \mathbf{13\%}$ 2. $4.375 = \mathbf{437.5\%}$ 3. $33.3 = \mathbf{3\ 330\%}$ 4. $0.09 = \mathbf{9\%}$

5. $0.88 = \mathbf{88\%}$

Convert the following percents to decimals:

1. $72\% = \mathbf{0.72}$ 2. $0.3\% = \mathbf{0.003}$ 3. $92.4\% = \mathbf{0.924}$ 4. $0.09\% = \mathbf{0.0009}$

5. $66.6\% = \mathbf{0.666}$

CONVERTING BETWEEN FRACTIONS AND PERCENT

Convert the following fractions to percent:

1. $\frac{3}{4} = 0.75 = \mathbf{75\%}$ 2. $\frac{28}{36} = 0.76 = \mathbf{76\%}$ 3. $\frac{55}{64} = 0.86 = \mathbf{86\%}$

4. $\frac{18}{20} = 0.9 = \mathbf{90\%}$ 5. $\frac{45}{50} = 0.9 = \mathbf{90\%}$

Convert the following percents to fractions.
Reduce the fractions to the lowest common denominator.

1. $40\% = \dfrac{40}{100} = \dfrac{2}{5}$ 2. $185\% = \dfrac{185}{100} = 1\dfrac{17}{20}$ 3. $75\% = \dfrac{75}{100} = \dfrac{3}{4}$

4. $66\% = \dfrac{66}{100} = \dfrac{33}{50}$ 5. $31\% = \dfrac{31}{100}$

CHAPTER 2

RATIOS

1. You have 15 carrots and 20 potatoes. What is the ratio of carrots to potatoes?

   15:20 or 15/20

2. Your term test has 40 questions. You answered 35 of them correctly. What is the ratio of questions answered correctly to the total number of questions? What is the ratio of incorrect answers to correct answers?

   Correct answers to total answers 35:40 or 35/40

   Incorrect answers to correct answers 5:35 or 5/35

3. Your cat has just had seven kittens. Three are black, two are white, one is grey, and one is orange. What is the ratio of black kittens to the total number of kittens? What is the ratio of white kittens to black kittens? What is the ratio of grey kittens to black kittens?

   Black kittens to total kittens 3:7 or 3/7

   White kittens to black kittens 2:3 or 2/3

   Grey kittens to black kittens 1:3 or 1/3

4. You are making fruit salad. The recipe calls for 2 cups of blueberries and 3 cups of strawberries. What is the ratio of blueberries to strawberries?

   Blueberries to strawberries 2:3 or 2/3

5. You are buying snacks for a party. You buy 12 bags of potato chips and 6 bags of taco chips. What is the ratio of taco chips to potato chips? What is the ratio of potato chips to the total number of bags of snacks?

   Taco chips to potato chips 6:12 or 6/12

   Potato chips to total bags of snacks 12:18 or 12/18

RATIO AND PROPORTION: MEANS = EXTREMES

1. The staffing ratio on your hospital unit is 1 nurse for each 6 patients. If there are 36 patients on the floor, how many nurses will there be?

   Ratio and Proportion: Means = Extremes

   The known ratio is 6 patients : 1 nurse
   The unknown ratio is 36 patients : X nurses
   The unknown ratio = the known ratio

$$\begin{array}{c} \downarrow\text{-means-}\downarrow \\ 36:X \quad = \quad 6:1 \\ \uparrow\text{---extremes---}\uparrow \end{array}$$

means = 6*X*
extremes = 36
means = extremes
6*X* = 36
X = 6
There will be 6 nurses.

2. You are making a stew. The recipe calls for 5 carrots for each potato that you put in. You decide to put in 15 carrots. How many potatoes will you put in?

Ratio and Proportion: Means = Extremes

The known ratio is 5 carrots : 1 potato
The unknown ratio is 15 carrots : *X* potatoes
The unknown ratio = the known ratio

$$\begin{array}{c} \downarrow\text{-means-}\downarrow \\ 15:X \quad = \quad 5:1 \\ \uparrow\text{---extremes---}\uparrow \end{array}$$

means = 5*X*
extremes = 15
means = extremes
5*X* = 15
X = 3
There will be 3 potatoes.

3. The pet store usually has 3 dogs for every 2 cats in the store. If there are 21 dogs, how many cats are there?

Ratio and Proportion: Means = Extremes

The known ratio is 3 dogs : 2 cats
The unknown ratio is 21 dogs : *X* cats
The unknown ratio = the known ratio

$$\begin{array}{c} \downarrow\text{-means-}\downarrow \\ 21:X \quad = \quad 3:2 \\ \uparrow\text{---extremes---}\uparrow \end{array}$$

means = 3*X*
extremes = 42
means = extremes
3*X* = 42
X = 14
There will be 14 cats.

4. The magazine has 5 pages of advertising for every 3 pages of news articles. If the magazine has 35 pages of advertising, how many pages of news articles does it have?

Ratio and Proportion: Means = Extremes

The known ratio is 5 ad pages : 3 news pages
The unknown ratio is 35 ad pages : *X* news pages
The unknown ratio = the known ratio

$$\begin{array}{c} \downarrow\text{-means-}\downarrow \\ 35:X \quad = \quad 5:3 \\ \uparrow\text{---extremes---}\uparrow \end{array}$$

means = 5X
extremes = 105
means = extremes
5X = 105
X = 21
There will be 21 pages of news.

5. The radio station plays 7 commercials for every 2 songs that it plays. If it plays 6 songs in an hour, how many commercials will it play?

Ratio and Proportion: Means = Extremes

The known ratio is 2 songs : 7 commercials
The unknown ratio is 6 songs : X commercials
The unknown ratio = the known ratio

$$\downarrow\text{-means-}\downarrow$$
$$6:X \;=\; 2:7$$
$$\uparrow\text{---extremes---}\uparrow$$

means = 2X
extremes = 42
means = extremes
2X = 42
X = 21
There will be 21 commercials.

RATIO AND PROPORTION: CROSS MULTIPLICATION OF FRACTIONS

You are making a fruit punch for a minor hockey league banquet. The original recipe calls for 1 000 ml of cranberry cocktail, 750 ml of white grape juice, 500 ml of pineapple juice, 125 ml of lemon juice and 750 ml of soda water. This will make 3 125 ml of punch. You estimate that you will need 25 000 ml for the banquet.

1. How many ml of cranberry cocktail will you need?

Ratio and Proportion: Cross Multiplication of Fractions

Known ratio is 1 000 ml in 3 125 ml $= \dfrac{1\,000}{3\,125}$

Unknown ratio is X ml in 25 000 ml $= \dfrac{X}{25\,000}$

Unknown ratio = Known ratio

$$\frac{X}{25\,000} = \frac{1\,000}{3\,125}$$

Cross Multiply

$$\frac{X}{25\,000} \;\nwarrow\nearrow\; \frac{1\,000}{3\,125} \;\swarrow\searrow$$

3 125X = 25 000 000
X = 8 000
You will need 8 000 ml of cranberry cocktail.

2. How many ml of white grape juice will you need?

Ratio and Proportion: Multiplication of Fractions

Known ratio is 750 ml in 3 125 ml $= \dfrac{750}{3\,125}$

Unknown ratio is X ml in 25 000 ml $= \dfrac{X}{25\,000}$

Unknown ratio = Known ratio

$$\frac{X}{25\,000} = \frac{750}{3\,125}$$

Cross Multiply

$$\frac{X}{25\,000} \nwarrow \nearrow \frac{750}{3\,125}$$
$$\swarrow \searrow$$

$3\,125X = 18\,750\,000$
$X = 6\,000$
You will need 6 000 ml of white grape juice.

3.   How many ml of pineapple juice will you need?

Ratio and Proportion: Cross Multiplication of Fractions

Known ratio is 500 ml in 3 125 ml = $\dfrac{500}{3\,125}$

Unknown ratio is X ml in 25 000 ml = $\dfrac{X}{25\,000}$

Unknown ratio = Known ratio

$$\frac{X}{25\,000} = \frac{500}{3\,125}$$

Cross Multiply

$$\frac{X}{25\,000} \nwarrow \nearrow \frac{500}{3\,125}$$
$$\swarrow \searrow$$

$3\,125X = 12\,500\,000$
$X = 4\,000$
You will need 4 000 ml of pineapple juice.

4.   How many ml of lemon juice will you need?

Ratio and Proportion: Cross Multiplication of Fractions

Known ratio is 125 ml in 3 125 ml = $\dfrac{125}{3\,125}$

Unknown ratio is X ml in 25 000 ml = $\dfrac{X}{25\,000}$

Unknown ratio = Known ratio

$$\frac{X}{25\,000} = \frac{125}{3\,125}$$

Cross Multiply

$$\frac{X}{25\,000} \nwarrow \nearrow \frac{125}{3\,125}$$
$$\swarrow \searrow$$

$3\,125X = 3\,125\,000$
$X = 1\,000$
You will need 1 000 ml of lemon juice.

5.   There are 500 ml of lemon juice in each bottle. How many bottles of lemon juice will you need?

Ratio and Proportion: Cross Multiplication of Fractions

Known ratio is 500 ml in 1 bottle = $\dfrac{500}{1}$

Unknown ratio is 1 000 ml in X bottles = $\dfrac{1\,000}{X}$

Unknown ratio = Known ratio

$$\frac{1\,000}{X} = \frac{500}{1}$$

Cross Multiply

$$\frac{1\,000}{X} \diagdown \diagup \frac{500}{1}$$

$500X = 1\,000$

$X = 2$

You will need 2 bottles of lemon juice.

CHAPTER 4

Convert the following values within the metric system.

1.   750 mg = <u>0.75</u> g

2.   2 L = <u>2 000</u> ml

3.   5 kg = <u>5 000</u> g

4.   1.5 g = <u>1 500</u> mg

5.   500 mg = <u>0.005</u> kg

6.   200 μg = <u>0.2</u> mg

Convert these 12-hour clock times to 24-hour clock times.

1.   4 pm <u>1600 hrs</u>

2.   3:15 am <u>0315 hrs</u>

3.   2:45 am <u>0245 hrs</u>

4.   11:40 pm <u>2340 hrs</u>

5.   11:40 am <u>1140 hrs</u>

Convert these 24-hour clock times to 12-hour clock times.

6.   0430 <u>4:30 am</u>

7.   1545 <u>3:30 pm</u>

8.   1910 <u>7:10 pm</u>

9.   0800 <u>8 am</u>

10. 1240 <u>1240 pm</u>

CHAPTER 8

ORAL SOLIDS

1.   *Ampicillin 750 mg tonight, then 500 mg QID for 10 days.* Stock **ampicillin 250 mg capsules.**

     How many capsules will you give tonight?

     <u> *3 capsules* </u>

Ratio and Proportion: Means = Extremes	**Ratio and Proportion: Cross Multiplication of Fractions**	**Formula**
The known ratio is 250 mg : 1 cap The unknown ratio is 750 mg : A cap	Known ratio is 250 mg in 1 cap $\dfrac{250}{1}$	$\dfrac{\text{Dose } \textbf{D}\text{esired (mg)}}{\text{Dose on } \textbf{H}\text{and (mg)}}$ $\times \textbf{S}\text{tock (pills)} = \textbf{A}\text{mount}$
↓-means-↓ 750 : A = 250 : 1 ↑----extremes-----↑	Unknown ratio is 750 mg in A cap $\dfrac{750}{A}$	or $\dfrac{\textbf{D}}{\textbf{H}} \times \textbf{S} = \textbf{A}$
Means = Extremes	$\dfrac{750 \text{ mg}}{A \text{ capsules}} \nwarrow \nearrow \dfrac{250 \text{ mg}}{1 \text{ capsule}}$	Dose **D**esired is 750 mg Dose on **H**and is 250 **S**tock is 1 capsule
250A = 750	250A = 750	$\dfrac{750 \text{ mg}}{250 \text{ mg}} \times 1 \text{ capsule} = \textbf{A}$
A = 3 capsules	A = 3 capsules	A = 3 capsules

How many capsules per dose will you give tomorrow? _2 capsules_

Ratio and Proportion: Means = Extremes	**Ratio and Proportion: Cross Multiplication of Fractions**	**Formula**
The known ratio is 250 mg : 1 cap The unknown ratio is 500 mg : A cap	Known ratio is 250 mg in 1 cap $\dfrac{250}{1}$	$\dfrac{\text{Dose } \textbf{D}\text{esired (mg)}}{\text{Dose on } \textbf{H}\text{and (mg)}}$ $\times \textbf{S}\text{tock (pills)} = \textbf{A}\text{mount}$
↓-means-↓ 500 : A = 250 : 1 ↑---extremes-----↑	Unknown ratio is 500 mg in A cap $\dfrac{500}{A}$	or $\dfrac{\textbf{D}}{\textbf{H}} \times \textbf{S} = \textbf{A}$
Means = Extremes	$\dfrac{500 \text{ mg}}{A \text{ capsules}} \nwarrow \nearrow \dfrac{250 \text{ mg}}{1 \text{ capsule}}$	Dose **D**esired is 500 mg Dose on **H**and is 250 **S**tock is 1 capsule
250A = 500	250A = 500	$\dfrac{500 \text{ mg}}{250 \text{ mg}} \times 1 \text{ capsule} = \textbf{A}$
A = 2 capsules	A = 2 capsules	A = 2 capsules

2. *Digoxin 0.125 mg OD*. Stock **Digoxin 0.25 mg** tablets. How many tablets will you give?

   1/2 tablet

Ratio and Proportion: Means = Extremes	**Ratio and Proportion: Cross Multiplication of Fractions**	**Formula**
The known ratio is 0.25 mg : 1 tab The unknown ratio is 0.125 mg : A tab	Known ratio is 0.25 mg in 1 tab $\dfrac{0.25}{1}$	$\dfrac{\text{Dose } \textbf{D}\text{esired (mg)}}{\text{Dose on } \textbf{H}\text{and (mg)}}$ $\times \textbf{S}\text{tock (pills)} = \textbf{A}\text{mount}$
↓-means-↓ 0.125 : A = 0.25 : 1 ↑-----extremes------↑	Unknown ratio is 0.125 mg in A tab $\dfrac{0.125}{A}$	or $\dfrac{\textbf{D}}{\textbf{H}} \times \textbf{S} = \textbf{A}$
Means = Extremes	$\dfrac{0.125 \text{ mg}}{A \text{ tablet}} \nwarrow \nearrow \dfrac{0.25 \text{ mg}}{1 \text{ tablet}}$	Dose **D**esired is 0.125 mg Dose on **H**and is 0.25 mg **S**tock is 1 tablet
0.25A = 0.125	0.25A = 0.125 A = 1/2 tablet	$\dfrac{0.125 \text{ mg}}{0.25 \text{ mg}} \times 1 \text{ tablet} = \textbf{A}$
A = 1/2 tablet		A = 1/2 tablet

3. *Gravol (dimenhydrinate) 75 mg Q4H PRN.* Stock **Gravol 50 mg tablets.**
   How many tablets will you give?

   $1\frac{1}{2}$

Ratio and Proportion: Means = Extremes	**Ratio and Proportion: Cross Multiplication of Fractions**	**Formula**
The known ratio is 50 mg : 1 tab The unknown ratio is 75 mg : A tab ↓-means-↓ 75 : A = 50 : 1 ↑---extremes----↑ Means = Extremes 50A = 75 A = 1 1/2 tablet	Known ratio is 50 mg in 1 tablet $\frac{50}{1}$ Unknown ratio is 75 mg in A tablets $\frac{75}{A}$ $\frac{75\ mg}{A\ tablet}$ ↖↗ $\frac{50\ mg}{1\ tablet}$ ↙↘ 50A = 75 A = 1 1/2 tablet	$\dfrac{\text{Dose \textbf{D}esired (mg)}}{\text{Dose on \textbf{H}and (mg)}}$ $\times$ **S**tock (pills) = **A**mount or $\dfrac{\textbf{D}}{\textbf{H}} \times \textbf{S} = \textbf{A}$ Dose **D**esired is 75 mg Dose on **H**and is 50 mg **S**tock is 1 tablet $\dfrac{75\ mg}{50\ mg} \times 1$ tablet = **A** A = 1 1/2 tablet

4. *Trazodone 25 mg QHS.* Stock **trazodone 50 mg tablets.**
   How many tablets will you give?

   1/2 tablet

Ratio and Proportion: Means = Extremes	**Ratio and Proportion: Cross Multiplication of Fractions**	**Formula**
The known ratio is 50 mg : 1 tab The unknown ratio is 25 mg : A tab ↓-means-↓ 25 : A = 50 : 1 ↑---extremes----↑ Means = Extremes 50A = 5 A = 1/2 tablet	Known ratio is 50 mg in 1 tablet $\frac{50}{1}$ Unknown ratio is 75 mg in A tablets $\frac{25}{A}$ $\frac{25\ mg}{A\ tablet}$ ↖↗ $\frac{50\ mg}{1\ tablet}$ ↙↘ 50A = 25 A = 1/2 tablet	$\dfrac{\text{Dose \textbf{D}esired (mg)}}{\text{Dose on \textbf{H}and (mg)}}$ $\times$ **S**tock (pills) = **A**mount or $\dfrac{\textbf{D}}{\textbf{H}} \times \textbf{S} = \textbf{A}$ Dose **D**esired is 25 mg Dose on **H**and is 50 mg **S**tock is 1 tablet $\dfrac{25\ mg}{50\ mg} \times 1$ tablet = **A** A = 1/2 tablet

5. *Cardizem (diltiazem) 90 mg BID.* Stock **Cardizem 30 mg tablets.**
   How many tablets will you give?

   3

Ratio and Proportion: Means = Extremes	**Ratio and Proportion: Cross Multiplication of Fractions**	**Formula**
The known ratio is 30 mg : 1 tab The unknown ratio is 90 mg : A tab ↓-means-↓ 90 : A = 30 : 1 ↑---extremes----↑ Means = Extremes 30A = 90 A = 3 tablets	Known ratio is 30 mg in 1 tablet $\frac{30}{1}$ Unknown ratio is 90 mg in A tablets $\frac{90}{A}$ $\frac{90\ mg}{A\ tablet}$ ↖↗ $\frac{30\ mg}{1\ tablet}$ ↙↘ 30A = 90 A = 3 tablets	$\dfrac{\text{Dose \textbf{D}esired (mg)}}{\text{Dose on \textbf{H}and (mg)}}$ $\times$ **S**tock (pills) = **A**mount or $\dfrac{\textbf{D}}{\textbf{H}} \times \textbf{S} = \textbf{A}$ Dose **D**esired is 90 mg Dose on **H**and is 30 mg **S**tock is 1 tablet $\dfrac{90\ mg}{30\ mg} \times 1$ tablet = **A** A = 3 tablets

ORAL LIQUIDS

The doctor's order reads *Tylenol (acetaminophen) 160 mg po Q4H PRN*. How many ml will you give?

1.   Stock **Tylenol 80 mg/0.8 ml**
     How many ml will you give?

     _____*1.6 ml*_____

Ratio and Proportion: Means = Extremes	**Ratio and Proportion: Cross Multiplication of Fractions**	**Formula**
The known ratio is 80 mg : 0.8 ml	Known ratio is 80 mg in	$\dfrac{\text{Dose } \mathbf{D}\text{esired (mg)}}{\text{Dose on } \mathbf{H}\text{and (mg)}}$
The unknown ratio is 160 mg : A ml	0.8 ml $\dfrac{80}{0.8}$	$\times \, \mathbf{S}\text{tock (pills)} = \mathbf{A}\text{mount}$
↓-means-↓ 160 : A = 80 : 0.8 ↑-----extremes-----↑	Unknown ratio is 160 mg in A ml $\dfrac{160}{A}$	or $\dfrac{\mathbf{D}}{\mathbf{H}} \times \mathbf{S} = \mathbf{A}$
Means = Extremes	$\dfrac{160 \text{ mg}}{\text{A ml}} \nwarrow \nearrow \dfrac{80 \text{ mg}}{0.8 \text{ ml}}$	Dose **D**esired is 160 mg Dose on **H**and is 80 mg **S**tock is 0.8 ml
80A = 128	80A = 128	$\dfrac{160 \text{ mg}}{80 \text{ mg}} \times 0.8 \text{ ml} = \mathbf{A}$
A = 1.6 ml	A = 1.6 ml	A = 1.6 ml

2.   Stock **Tylenol 80 mg/2.5 ml**
     How many ml will you give?

     _____*5 ml*_____

Ratio and Proportion: Means = Extremes	**Ratio and Proportion: Cross Multiplication of Fractions**	**Formula**
The known ratio is 80 mg : 2.5 ml	Known ratio is 80 mg in	$\dfrac{\text{Dose } \mathbf{D}\text{esired (mg)}}{\text{Dose on } \mathbf{H}\text{and (mg)}}$
The unknown ratio is 160 mg : A ml	2.5 ml $\dfrac{80}{2.5}$	$\times \, \mathbf{S}\text{tock (pills)} = \mathbf{A}\text{mount}$
↓-means-↓ 160 : A = 80 : 2.5 ↑----extremes----↑	Unknown ratio is 160 mg in A ml $\dfrac{160}{A}$	or $\dfrac{\mathbf{D}}{\mathbf{H}} \times \mathbf{S} = \mathbf{A}$
Means = Extremes	$\dfrac{160 \text{ mg}}{\text{A ml}} \nwarrow \nearrow \dfrac{80 \text{ mg}}{2.5 \text{ ml}}$	Dose **D**esired is 160 mg Dose on **H**and is 80 mg **S**tock is 2.5 ml
80A = 400	80A = 400	$\dfrac{160 \text{ mg}}{80 \text{ mg}} \times 2.5 \text{ ml} = \mathbf{A}$
A = 5 ml	A = 5 ml	A = 5 ml

3. Stock Tylenol 80 mg/5 ml
    How many ml will you give? _____ *10 ml* _____

Ratio and Proportion: Means = Extremes

The known ratio is
80 mg : 5 ml
The unknown ratio is
160 mg : A ml

↓-means-↓
160 : A = 80 : 5
↑---extremes-----↑

Means = Extremes

80A = 800

A = 10 ml

Ratio and Proportion: Cross Multiplication of Fractions

Known ratio is 80 mg in
5 ml $\dfrac{80}{5}$

Unknown ratio is 160 mg in
A ml $\dfrac{160}{A}$

$\dfrac{160\ mg}{A\ ml}$ ↖ ↗ $\dfrac{80\ mg}{5\ ml}$
        ↙ ↘

80A = 800

A = 10 ml

Formula

$\dfrac{\text{Dose \textbf{D}esired (mg)}}{\text{Dose on \textbf{H}and (mg)}}$
   $\times$ **S**tock (pills) = **A**mount

or $\dfrac{D}{H} \times S = A$

Dose **D**esired is 160 mg
Dose on **H**and is 80 mg
Stock is 5 ml

$\dfrac{160\ mg}{80\ mg} \times 5\ ml = A$

A = 10 ml

4. Stock Tylenol 120 mg/5ml
    How many ml will you give? _____ *6.7 ml* _____

Ratio and Proportion: Means = Extremes

The known ratio is
120 mg : 5 ml
The unknown ratio is
160 mg : A ml

↓-means-↓
160 : A = 120 : 5
↑----extremes-----↑

Means = Extremes

120A = 800

A = 6.7 ml

Ratio and Proportion: Cross Multiplication of Fractions

Known ratio is 120 mg in
5 ml $\dfrac{120}{5}$

Unknown ratio is 160 mg in
A ml $\dfrac{160}{A}$

$\dfrac{160\ mg}{A\ ml}$ ↖ ↗ $\dfrac{120\ mg}{5\ ml}$
        ↙ ↘

120A = 800

A = 6.7 ml

Formula

$\dfrac{\text{Dose \textbf{D}esired (mg)}}{\text{Dose on \textbf{H}and (mg)}}$
   $\times$ **S**tock (pills) = **A**mount

or $\dfrac{D}{H} \times S = A$

Dose **D**esired is 160 mg
Dose on **H**and is 120 mg
Stock is 5 ml

$\dfrac{160\ mg}{120\ mg} \times 5\ ml = A$

A = 6.7 ml

5. Stock Tylenol 160 mg/5 ml
    How many ml will you give? _____ *5 ml* _____

Ratio and Proportion: Means = Extremes

The known ratio is
160 mg : 5 ml
The unknown ratio is
160 mg : A ml

↓-means-↓
160 : A = 160 : 5
↑---extremes-----↑

Means = Extremes

160A = 800

A = 5 ml

Ratio and Proportion: Cross Multiplication of Fractions

Known ratio is 160 mg in
5 ml $\dfrac{160}{5}$

Unknown ratio is 160 mg in
A ml $\dfrac{160}{A}$

$\dfrac{160\ mg}{A\ ml}$ ↖ ↗ $\dfrac{160\ mg}{5\ ml}$
        ↙ ↘

160A = 800

A = 5 ml

Formula

$\dfrac{\text{Dose \textbf{D}esired (mg)}}{\text{Dose on \textbf{H}and (mg)}}$
   $\times$ **S**tock (pills) = **A**mount

or $\dfrac{D}{H} \times S = A$

Dose **D**esired is 160 mg
Dose on **H**and is 160 mg
Stock is 5 ml

$\dfrac{160\ mg}{160\ mg} \times 5\ ml = A$

A = 5 ml

CHAPTER 9

LIQUID PREPARATIONS

1. The doctor's order reads *Demerol (meperidine) 75 mg IM Q3H PRN.* The label on the ampoule reads **Demerol 100 mg/ml.** How much Demerol will you give?

   <u>   0.75 ml   </u>

Ratio and Proportion: Means = Extremes	**Ratio and Proportion: Cross Multiplication of Fractions**	**Formula**
Known ratio 100 mg : 1ml	Known ratio $\dfrac{100\ mg}{1\ ml}$	$\dfrac{Dose\ \textbf{D}esired}{Dose\ on\ \textbf{H}and} \times \textbf{S}tock$
Unknown ratio 75 mg : A ml		$= \textbf{A}mount$
75 mg : A ml : 100 mg : 1 ml	Unknown ratio $\dfrac{75\ mg}{A\ ml}$	$\dfrac{\textbf{D}}{\textbf{H}} \times \textbf{S} = \textbf{A}$
100A = 75	$\dfrac{75\ mg}{A\ ml} \nwarrow \nearrow \dfrac{100\ mg}{1\ ml}$	**D** is 75 mg
A = .75 ml	$\swarrow \searrow$	**H** is 100 mg
	100A = 75	**S** is 1 ml
	A = .75 ml	$\dfrac{75\ mg}{100\ mg} \times 1\ ml = \textbf{A}\ ml$
		A = .75 ml

2. The doctor's order reads *Largactil (chlorpromazine) 150 mg IM TID.* The label reads **Largactil 50 mg/2ml.** How much Largactil will you give?

   <u>   6 ml   </u>

Ratio and Proportion: Means = Extremes	**Ratio and Proportion: Cross Multiplication of Fractions**	**Formula**
Known ratio 50 mg : 2 ml	Known ratio $\dfrac{50\ mg}{2\ ml}$	$\dfrac{Dose\ \textbf{D}esired}{Dose\ on\ \textbf{H}and} \times \textbf{S}tock$
Unknown ratio 150 mg : A ml		$= \textbf{A}mount$
150 mg : A ml : 50 mg : 2 ml	Unknown ratio $\dfrac{150\ mg}{A\ ml}$	$\dfrac{\textbf{D}}{\textbf{H}} \times \textbf{S} = \textbf{A}$
50A = 300	$\dfrac{150\ mg}{A\ ml} \nwarrow \nearrow \dfrac{50\ mg}{2\ ml}$	**D** is 150 mg
A = 6 ml	$\swarrow \searrow$	**H** is 50 mg
	50A = 300	**S** is 2 ml
	A = 6 ml	$\dfrac{150\ mg}{50\ mg} \times 2\ ml = \textbf{A}\ ml$
		A = 6 ml

3.   The doctor's order reads *Zantac (ranitidine) 50 mg IV BID*. The label reads **Zantac 25 mg/ml.** How much Zantac will you give?

_____*2 ml*_____

Ratio and Proportion: Means = Extremes	Ratio and Proportion: Cross Multiplication of Fractions	Formula
Known ratio 25 mg : 1 ml Unknown ratio 50 mg : A ml 50 mg : A ml : 25 mg : 1 ml 25A = 50 A = 2 ml	Known ratio $\dfrac{25\ mg}{1\ ml}$ Unknown ratio $\dfrac{50\ mg}{A\ ml}$ $\dfrac{50\ mg}{A\ ml} \nwarrow \nearrow \dfrac{25\ mg}{1\ ml}$ $\swarrow \searrow$ 25A = 50 A = 2 ml	$\dfrac{\text{Dose \textbf{D}esired}}{\text{Dose on \textbf{H}and}} \times \textbf{S}\text{tock}$ $= \textbf{A}\text{mount}$ $\dfrac{\textbf{D}}{\textbf{H}} \times \textbf{S} = \textbf{A}$ **D** is 50 mg **H** is 25 mg **S** is 1 ml $\dfrac{50\ mg}{25\ mg} \times 1\ ml = \textbf{A}\ ml$ A = 2 ml

4.   The doctor's order reads *Valium (diazepam) 2.5 mg IV push Stat*. The label reads **Valium 5 mg/ml.** How much Valium will you give?

_____*0.5 ml*_____

Ratio and Proportion: Means = Extremes	Ratio and Proportion: Cross Multiplication of Fractions	Formula
Known ratio 5 mg : 1 ml Unknown ratio 2.5 mg : A ml 2.5 mg : A ml : 5 mg : 1 ml 5A = 2.5 A = 0.5 ml	Known ratio $\dfrac{5\ mg}{1\ ml}$ Unknown ratio $\dfrac{2.5\ mg}{A\ ml}$ $\dfrac{2.5\ mg}{A\ ml} \nwarrow \nearrow \dfrac{5\ mg}{1\ ml}$ $\swarrow \searrow$ 5A = 2.5 A = 0.5 ml	$\dfrac{\text{Dose \textbf{D}esired}}{\text{Dose on \textbf{H}and}} \times \textbf{S}\text{tock}$ $= \textbf{A}\text{mount}$ $\dfrac{\textbf{D}}{\textbf{H}} \times \textbf{S} = \textbf{A}$ **D** is 2.5 mg **H** is 5 mg **S** is 1 ml $\dfrac{2.5\ mg}{5\ mg} \times 1\ ml = \textbf{A}\ ml$ A = 0.5 ml

5.   The doctor's order reads *Gravol (dimenhydrinate) 12.5 mg IM Q4H PRN*. the label reads **Gravol 50 mg/ml.** How much Gravol will you give?

_____*0.25*_____

Ratio and Proportion: Means = Extremes	Ratio and Proportion: Cross Multiplication of Fractions	Formula
Known ratio 50 mg : 1 ml Unknown ratio 12.5 mg : A ml 12.5 mg : A ml : 50 mg : 1 ml 50A = 12.5 A = 0.25 ml	Known ratio $\dfrac{50\ mg}{1\ ml}$ Unknown ratio $\dfrac{12.5\ mg}{A\ ml}$ $\dfrac{12.5\ mg}{A\ ml} \nwarrow \nearrow \dfrac{50\ mg}{1\ ml}$ $\swarrow \searrow$ 50A = 12.5 A = 0.25 ml	$\dfrac{\text{Dose \textbf{D}esired}}{\text{Dose on \textbf{H}and}} \times \textbf{S}\text{tock}$ $= \textbf{A}\text{mount}$ $\dfrac{\textbf{D}}{\textbf{H}} \times \textbf{S} = \textbf{A}$ **D** is 12.5 mg **H** is 50 mg **S** is 1 ml $\dfrac{12.5\ mg}{50\ mg} \times 1\ ml = \textbf{A}\ ml$ A = 0.25 ml

RECONSTITUTING POWDERS

1. The doctor's order reads *Tazidime (ceftazidime) 750 mg IV Q8H.* The label on the vial reads **Tazidime 2 g.** The reconstitution table reads as follows:

Vial Size	Diluent	Volume to be Added to Vial(ml)	Approximate Available Volume (ml)	Nominal Concentration (mg/ml)
2 g	Sterile water for injection	10	11.2	180

How much of the solution will you give for each dose?

        4 ml

How many doses will this vial provide?

$$\frac{11.2\ ml}{4\ ml} = 2\ doses$$

Ratio and Proportion: Means = Extremes

Known ratio   180 mg : 1 ml
Unknown ratio   750 mg : A ml

750 mg : A ml : 180 mg : 1 ml

180A = 750

A = 4 ml

Ratio and Proportion: Cross Multiplication of Fractions

Known ratio $\dfrac{180\ mg}{1\ ml}$

Unknown ratio $\dfrac{750\ mg}{A\ ml}$

$\dfrac{750\ mg}{A\ ml} \nwarrow \nearrow \dfrac{180\ mg}{1\ ml}$
$ \swarrow \searrow$

180A = 750

A = 4 ml

Formula

$$\frac{\text{Dose } \mathbf{D}\text{esired}}{\text{Dose on } \mathbf{H}\text{and}} \times \mathbf{S}\text{tock}$$

$$= \mathbf{A}\text{mount}$$

$$\frac{\mathbf{D}}{\mathbf{H}} \times \mathbf{S} = \mathbf{A}$$

D is 750 mg
H is 180 mg
S is 1 ml

$$\frac{750\ mg}{180\ mg} \times 1\ ml = \mathbf{A}\ ml$$

A = 4 ml

2. The doctor's order reads *cefotetan 600 mg IV Q12H.* The label on the vial reads **cefotetan 1 gm.** The label also states that the vial should be diluted with 10 ml of sterile water for injection yielding a concentration of 95 mg/ml. How much solution will you give for each dose?

        6.3 ml

Ratio and Proportion: Means = Extremes

Known ratio   95 mg : 1 ml
Unknown ratio   600 mg : A ml

600 mg : A ml : 95 mg : 1 ml

95A = 600

A = 6.3 ml

Ratio and Proportion: Cross Multiplication of Fractions

Known ratio $\dfrac{95\ mg}{1\ ml}$

Unknown ratio $\dfrac{600\ mg}{A\ ml}$

$\dfrac{600\ mg}{A\ ml} \nwarrow \nearrow \dfrac{95\ mg}{1\ ml}$
$ \swarrow \searrow$

95A = 600

A = 6.3 ml

Formula

$$\frac{\text{Dose } \mathbf{D}\text{esired}}{\text{Dose on } \mathbf{H}\text{and}} \times \mathbf{S}\text{tock}$$

$$= \mathbf{A}\text{mount}$$

$$\frac{\mathbf{D}}{\mathbf{H}} \times \mathbf{S} = \mathbf{A}$$

D is 600 mg
H is 95 mg
S is 1 ml

$$\frac{600\ mg}{95\ mg} \times 1\ ml = \mathbf{A}\ ml$$

A = 6.3 ml

3. The doctor's order reads *Pipracil (piperacillin) 1 g IM Q6H*. The label on the vial reads **Pipracil 2 g.** The reconstitution directions on the label read: add 4 ml sterile water for injection. Approximate concentration 0.4 g/ml. How much will you give?

    NOTE: *Keep in mind that you are working in grams in this question rather than milligrams, but the calculation methods stay the same.*

    _____2.5 ml_____

Ratio and Proportion: Means = Extremes	Ratio and Proportion: Cross Multiplication of Fractions	Formula
Known ratio 0.4 g : 1 ml Unknown ratio 1 g : A ml 1 g : A ml : 0.4 g : 1 ml 0.4A = 1 A = .2.5 ml	Known ratio $\dfrac{0.4\ g}{1\ ml}$ Unknown ratio $\dfrac{1\ g}{A\ ml}$ $\dfrac{1\ g}{A\ ml} \nwarrow \nearrow \dfrac{0.4\ g}{1\ ml}$ $\qquad \swarrow \searrow$ 0.4 A = 1 A = 2.5 ml	$\dfrac{\text{Dose } \mathbf{D}\text{esired}}{\text{Dose on } \mathbf{H}\text{and}} \times \mathbf{S}\text{tock}$ $\qquad = \mathbf{A}\text{mount}$ $\dfrac{\mathbf{D}}{\mathbf{H}} \times \mathbf{S} = \mathbf{A}$ **D** is 1 g **H** is 0.4 g **S** is 1 ml $\dfrac{1\ g}{0.4\ g} \times 1\ ml = \mathbf{A}\ ml$ A = 2.5 ml

4. The doctor's order reads *Mefoxin (cefoxitin) 1.5 g IV Q8H*. You have **Mefoxin 1 g** vials and **Mefoxin 2 g** vials available. The reconstitution table is as follows:

Vial Size	Diluent	Volume to be Added to Vial (ml)	Approximate Available Volume (ml)	Nominal Concentration (mg/ml)
1 g	Sterile water for injection or 0.9% sodium chloride injection	10	10.5	95
2 g	Sterile water for injection or 0.9% sodium chloride injection	10	11.1	180

If you use two 1 g vials, how much solution will you draw up in total?

_____15.8 ml_____

NOTE: *Before calculating this problem, you must ensure that you are working in the same units. The dose of medication is in grams, the concentration is given to you in milligrams. You may convert the dose to milligrams or you may convert the concentration to grams. It is probably easier in this problem to convert the dose to milligrams. 1.5 g = 1 500 mg*

Ratio and Proportion: Means = Extremes

Known ratio   95 mg : 1 ml
Unknown ratio   1 500 mg : A ml

1 500 mg : A ml : 95 mg : 1 ml

95A = 1 500

A = 15.8 ml

Ratio and Proportion: Cross Multiplication of Fractions

Known ratio $\dfrac{95 \text{ mg}}{1 \text{ ml}}$

Unknown ratio $\dfrac{1\,500 \text{ mg}}{A \text{ ml}}$

$\dfrac{1\,500 \text{ mg}}{A \text{ ml}} \nwarrow \nearrow \dfrac{95 \text{ mg}}{1 \text{ ml}}$

95A = 1 500

A = 15.8 ml

Formula

$\dfrac{\text{Dose } \mathbf{D}\text{esired}}{\text{Dose on } \mathbf{H}\text{and}} \times \mathbf{S}\text{tock}$

    $= \mathbf{A}\text{mount}$

$\dfrac{\mathbf{D}}{\mathbf{H}} \times \mathbf{S} = \mathbf{A}$

D is 1 500 mg
H is 95 mg
S is 1 ml

$\dfrac{1\,500 \text{ mg}}{95 \text{ mg}} \times 1 \text{ ml} = \mathbf{A} \text{ ml}$

A = 15.8 ml

If you use the 2 g vial, how much solution will you draw up in total?

    8.3 ml

Ratio and Proportion: Means = Extremes

Known ratio   180 mg : 1 ml
Unknown ratio 1 500 mg : A ml

1 500 mg : A ml : 180 mg : 1 ml

180A = 1 500

A = 8.3 ml

Ratio and Proportion: Cross Multiplication of Fractions

Known ratio $\dfrac{180 \text{ mg}}{1 \text{ ml}}$

Unknown ratio $\dfrac{1\,500 \text{ mg}}{A \text{ ml}}$

$\dfrac{1\,500 \text{ mg}}{A \text{ ml}} \nwarrow \nearrow \dfrac{180 \text{ mg}}{1 \text{ ml}}$

180A = 1 500

A = 8.3 ml

Formula

$\dfrac{\text{Dose } \mathbf{D}\text{esired}}{\text{Dose on } \mathbf{H}\text{and}} \times \mathbf{S}\text{tock}$

    $= \mathbf{A}\text{mount}$

$\dfrac{\mathbf{D}}{\mathbf{H}} \times \mathbf{S} = \mathbf{A}$

D is 1 500 mg
H is 180 mg
S is 1 ml

$\dfrac{1\,500 \text{ mg}}{180 \text{ mg}} \times 1 \text{ ml} = \mathbf{A} \text{ ml}$

A = 8.3 ml

CHAPTER 12

IV FLOW AND DRIP RATES FOR MACRO TUBING

1. Doctor's order *D5W 1 200 ml IV Q8H*. Drip factor is 15. Calculate the drip rate.

Two-Step Method

Step 1
Flow rate: (ml/hr)

$\dfrac{\text{amount of fluid}}{\text{time in hours}} = \text{flow rate}$

$\dfrac{1\,200 \text{ ml}}{8 \text{ hr}} = 150 \text{ ml/hr}$

Step 2
Drip rate: (gtts/min)

$\dfrac{\text{flow rate}}{60} \times \text{drip factor} = \text{drip rate}$

$\dfrac{150}{60} \times 15 = 37.5 \text{ gtts/min}$

The drip rate is **38 gtts/min.**

One-Step Method

$$\frac{\text{amount of fluid} \times \text{drip factor}}{\text{time in hours} \times 60 \text{ minutes}} = \text{drip rate}$$

$$\frac{1\ 200 \text{ ml} \times 15 \text{ gtts/ml}}{8 \text{ hrs} \times 60 \text{ minutes}} = 37.5 \text{ gtts/min}$$

The drip rate is **38 gtts/min.**

2. Doctor's order reads *IV Ringer's Lactate 500 ml Q12H.* Drip factor is 10. Calculate the drip rate.

Two-Step Method

Step 1
Flow rate: (ml/hr)

$$\frac{\text{amount of fluid}}{\text{time in hours}} = \text{flow rate}$$

$$\frac{500 \text{ ml}}{12 \text{ hr}} = 42 \text{ ml/hr}$$

Step 2
Drip rate: (gtts/min)

$$\frac{\text{flow rate}}{60} \times \text{drip factor} = \text{drip rate}$$

$$\frac{42 \text{ ml/hr}}{60} \times 10 = 7 \text{ gtts/min}$$

The drip rate is **7 gtts/min.**

One-Step Method

$$\frac{\text{amount of fluid} \times \text{drip factor}}{\text{time in hours} \times 60 \text{ minutes}} = \text{drip rate}$$

$$\frac{500 \text{ ml} \times 10 \text{ gtts/ml}}{12 \text{ hrs} \times 60 \text{ minutes}} = 6.9 \text{ gtts/min}$$

The drip rate is **7 gtts/min.**

3. Doctor's order *IV 2/3 & 1/3 200 ml/hr for 12 hours, then 100 ml hr for 24 hours.* Drip factor is 12. Calculate both drip rates.

Drip rate: (gtts/min)

$$\frac{\text{flow rate} \times \text{drip factor}}{60} = \text{drip rate}$$

$$\frac{200 \text{ ml/hr} \times 12}{60} = 40 \text{ gtts/min}$$

The drip rate is **40 gtts/min for 12 hours.**

Drip rate: (gtts/min)

$$\frac{\text{flow rate} \times \text{drip factor}}{60} = \text{drip rate}$$

$$\frac{100 \text{ ml/hr} \times 12}{60} = 20 \text{ gtts/min}$$

The drip rate is **20 gtts/min for 24 hours.**

4. Doctor's order reads *IV NS 3 000 per day*. Drip factor is 15. Calculate the drip rate.

Two-Step Method

Step 1
Flow rate: (ml/hr)

$$\frac{\text{amount of fluid}}{\text{time in hours}} = \text{flow rate}$$

$$\frac{3\ 000\ \text{ml}}{24\ \text{hr}} = 125\ \text{ml/hr}$$

Step 2
Drip rate: (gtts/min)

$$\frac{\text{flow rate}}{60} \times \text{drip factor} = \text{drip rate}$$

$$\frac{125\ \text{ml/hr}}{60} \times 15 = 31.25\ \text{gtts/min}$$

The IV will run at **32 gtts/min.**

One-Step Method

$$\frac{\text{amount of fluid} \times \text{drip factor}}{\text{time in hours} \times 60\ \text{minutes}} = \text{drip rate}$$

$$\frac{3\ 000\ \text{ml} \times 15\ \text{gtts/ml}}{24\ \text{hrs} \times 60\ \text{minutes}} = 31.25\ \text{gtts/min}$$

The IV will run at **32 gtts/min.**

DRIP RATES FOR MICRO TUBING

1. Doctor's order reads *IV NS 300 ml/shift* (8-hour shift). Calculate the drip rate.

$$\frac{\text{amount of fluid (ml)}}{\text{time in hours}} = \text{flow rate (ml/hr)}$$

$$\frac{300}{8} = \textbf{37.5 gtts/min}$$

2. Doctor's order reads *IV D5W 400 ml Q8H*. Calculate the drip rate.

$$\frac{\text{amount of fluid (ml)}}{\text{time in hours}} = \text{flow rate (ml/hr)}$$

$$\frac{400}{8} = \textbf{50 gtts/min}$$

3. Doctor's order reads *IV Normosol M 1 litre Q24H*. Calculate the drip rate.

$$\frac{\text{amount of fluid (ml)}}{\text{time in hours}} = \text{flow rate (ml/hr)}$$

$$\frac{1\ 000}{24} = \textbf{42 gtts/min}$$

4. Doctor's order reads *IV 5% dextrose in normal saline 30 ml/hr*. Calculate the drip rate.

$$\frac{\text{amount of fluid (ml)}}{\text{time in hours}} = \text{flow rate (ml/hr)}$$

$$\frac{30}{1} = \textbf{30 gtts/min}$$

5. Doctor's order reads *IV D5W 400 ml Q12H.* Calculate the drip rate.

$$\frac{\text{amount of fluid (ml)}}{\text{time in hours}} = \text{flow rate (ml/hr)}$$

$$\frac{400}{12} = \textbf{33 gtts/min}$$

CHAPTER 13

DRIP RATE FOR INTERMITTENT IV MEDICATIONS

1. The doctor's order reads *ranitidine 50 mg IV QHS.* The label on the stock reads **ranitidine 50 mg in 2 ml.** You decide that you will further dilute it to 75 ml of fluid and administer it over 20 minutes. What is the drip rate?

$$\frac{\text{amount of solution (ml)} \times 60}{\text{time (minutes)}} = \text{flow rate} = \text{drip rate}$$

$$\frac{75 \times 60}{20} = 225 \text{ ml/hr} = \textbf{225 gtts/min}$$

2. The doctor's order reads *Solu-Medrol 125 mg IV Q6H.* When reconstituted, the strength is 125 mg/2 ml. You decide that you will further dilute it to 100 ml of fluid and administer it over 40 minutes. What is the drip rate?

$$\frac{\text{amount of solution (ml)} \times 60}{\text{time (minutes)}} = \text{flow rate} = \text{drip rate}$$

$$\frac{100 \times 60}{40} = 150 \text{ ml/hr} = \textbf{150 gtts/min}$$

3. The doctor's order reads *Kefzol (cefazolin) 1 g IV QID.* When reconstituted, the strength is 125 mg/2 ml. When reconstituted, the strength is 1 g/10 ml. You decide that you will further dilute it to 100 ml of fluid and administer it over 1 hour. What is the drip rate?

$$\frac{\text{amount of solution (ml)} \times 60}{\text{time (minutes)}} = \text{flow rate} = \text{drip rate}$$

$$\frac{100 \times 60}{60} = 100 \text{ ml/hr} = \textbf{100 gtts/min}$$

4. The doctor's order reads *gentamycin 40 mg IV Q8H.* The label on the stock reads **gentamycin 40 mg in 1 ml.** You decide that you will further dilute it to 50 ml of fluid and administer it over 45 minutes. What is the drip rate?

$$\frac{\text{amount of solution (ml)} \times 60}{\text{time (minutes)}} = \text{flow rate} = \text{drip rate}$$

$$\frac{50 \times 60}{45} = 67 \text{ ml/hr} = \textbf{67 gtts/min}$$

5. The doctor's order reads *dimenhydrinate 50 mg IV QHS.* The label on the stock reads **dimenhydrinate 50 mg in 1 ml.** You decide that you will further dilute it to 50 ml of fluid and administer it over 20 minutes. What is the drip rate?

$$\frac{\text{amount of solution (ml)} \times 60}{\text{time (minutes)}} = \text{flow rate} = \text{drip rate}$$

$$\frac{50 \times 60}{20} = 150 \text{ ml/hr} = \textbf{150 gtts/min}$$

CONTINUOUS INFUSION OF IV MEDICATIONS

1. Doctor's order *furosemide 4 mg/hr IV*. The bag we have mixed has a concentration of furosemide **100 mg/100 ml** of IV fluid. At what flow rate will you run the pump?

Ratio and Proportion: **Means = Extremes**	**Ratio and Proportion:** **Cross Multiplication of** **Fractions**	**Formula**
Known ratio 100 mg : 100 ml Unknown ratio 4 mg : A ml 4 mg : A ml : 100 mg : 100 ml Means = 100 × A = 100A Extremes = 4 × 100 = 400 Means = Extremes 100A = 400 A = 4 You will run the pump at **4 ml/hr**	Known ratio $\dfrac{100 \text{ mg}}{100 \text{ ml}}$ Unknown ratio $\dfrac{4 \text{ mg}}{A \text{ ml}}$ $\dfrac{4 \text{ mg}}{A \text{ ml}} \begin{smallmatrix}\nwarrow & \nearrow\\ \swarrow & \searrow\end{smallmatrix} \dfrac{100 \text{ mg}}{100 \text{ ml}}$ 100A = 400 A = 4 You will run the pump at **4 ml/hr**	$\dfrac{\text{Dose } \mathbf{D}\text{esired}}{\text{Dose on } \mathbf{H}\text{and}} \times \mathbf{S}\text{tock}$ $\quad = \mathbf{A}\text{mount}$ $\dfrac{\mathbf{D}}{\mathbf{H}} \times \mathbf{S} = \mathbf{A}$ **D** is 4 mg **H** is 100 mg **S** is 100 ml $\dfrac{4 \text{ mg}}{100 \text{ mg}} \times 100 \text{ ml} = \mathbf{A} \text{ ml}$ A = 4 ml You will run the pump at **4 ml/hr**

2. Doctor's order reads *lidocaine 2 mg/min IV*. Lidocaine comes in a premixed 250-ml bag with a concentration of **8 mg/ml**. At what flow rate will you run the pump?

Convert time from mg/min to mg/hour.

2 mg/min = 2 × 60 = 120 mg/hour

Ratio and Proportion: **Means = Extremes**	**Ratio and Proportion:** **Cross Multiplication of** **Fractions**	**Formula**
Known ratio 8 mg : 1 ml Unknown ratio 120 mg : A ml 120 mg : A ml : 8 mg : 1 ml Means = 8 × A = 8A Extremes = 120 × 1 = 120 Means = Extremes 8A = 120 A = 15 You will run the pump at **15 ml/hr**	Known ratio $\dfrac{8 \text{ mg}}{1 \text{ ml}}$ Unknown ratio $\dfrac{120 \text{ mg}}{A \text{ ml}}$ $\dfrac{120 \text{ mg}}{A \text{ ml}} \begin{smallmatrix}\nwarrow & \nearrow\\ \swarrow & \searrow\end{smallmatrix} \dfrac{8 \text{ mg}}{1 \text{ ml}}$ 8A = 120 A = 15 You will run the pump at **15 ml/hr**	$\dfrac{\text{Dose } \mathbf{D}\text{esired}}{\text{Dose on } \mathbf{H}\text{and}} \times \mathbf{S}\text{tock}$ $\quad = \mathbf{A}\text{mount}$ $\dfrac{\mathbf{D}}{\mathbf{H}} \times \mathbf{S} = \mathbf{A}$ **D** is 120 mg **H** is 8 mg **S** is 1 ml $\dfrac{120 \text{ mg}}{8 \text{ mg}} \times 1 \text{ ml} = \mathbf{A} \text{ ml}$ A = 15 ml You will run the pump at **15 ml/hr**

3. Doctor's order *Isuprel (isoproterenol) 5 mcg/min IV.* Manufacturer's directions state that **1 mg of Isuprel is to be added to a 250 ml bag of D5W.** At what flow rate will you run the pump?

    Convert mcg/min to mg/min.

    5 mcg = 0.005 mg/min

    Convert time from mg/min to mg/hour.

    0.005 mg/min = 0.005 × 60 = 0.3 mg/hr

Ratio and Proportion: Means = Extremes	**Ratio and Proportion: Cross Multiplication of Fractions**	**Formula**
Known ratio 1 mg : 250 ml	Known ratio $\dfrac{1 \text{ mg}}{250 \text{ ml}}$	$\dfrac{\text{Dose } \mathbf{D}\text{esired}}{\text{Dose on } \mathbf{H}\text{and}} \times \mathbf{S}\text{tock}$
Unknown ratio 0.3 mg : A ml		$= \mathbf{A}\text{mount}$
0.3 mg : A ml : 1 mg : 250 ml	Unknown ratio $\dfrac{0.3 \text{ mg}}{A \text{ ml}}$	$\dfrac{\mathbf{D}}{\mathbf{H}} \times \mathbf{S} = \mathbf{A}$
Means = 1 × A = A	$\dfrac{0.3 \text{ mg}}{A \text{ ml}} \nwarrow \nearrow \dfrac{1 \text{ mg}}{250 \text{ ml}}$	**D** is 0.3 mg
Extremes = 0.3 × 250 = 75	$\swarrow \searrow$	**H** is 1 mg
		S is 250 ml
Means = Extremes	A = 75	$\dfrac{0.3 \text{ mg}}{1 \text{ mg}} \times 250 \text{ ml} = \mathbf{A} \text{ ml}$
A = 75	You will run the pump at	
You will run the pump at **75 ml/hr**	**75 ml/hr**	A = 75 ml
		You will run the pump at **75 ml/hr**

4. Doctor's order *nitroglycerine 400 mcg/min IV.* The premixed bag contains a concentration of **0.2 mg/ml.** At what flow rate will you run the pump?

    Convert mcg/min to mg/min.
    400 mcg = 0.4 mg/min

    Convert time from mg/min to mg/hr.
    0.4 mg/min = 0.4 × 60 = 24 mg/hr

Ratio and Proportion: Means = Extremes	**Ratio and Proportion: Cross Multiplication of Fractions**	**Formula**
Known ratio 0.2 mg : 1 ml	Known ratio $\dfrac{0.2 \text{ mg}}{1 \text{ ml}}$	$\dfrac{\text{Dose } \mathbf{D}\text{esired}}{\text{Dose on } \mathbf{H}\text{and}} \times \mathbf{S}\text{tock}$
Unknown ratio 24 mg : A ml		$= \mathbf{A}\text{mount}$
24 mg : A ml : 0.2 mg : 1 ml	Unknown ratio $\dfrac{24 \text{ mg}}{A \text{ ml}}$	$\dfrac{\mathbf{D}}{\mathbf{H}} \times \mathbf{S} = \mathbf{A}$
Means = 0.2 × A = 0.2A	$\dfrac{24 \text{ mg}}{A \text{ ml}} \nwarrow \nearrow \dfrac{0.2 \text{ mg}}{1 \text{ ml}}$	**D** is 24 mg
Extremes = 24 × 1 = 24	$\swarrow \searrow$	**H** is 0.2 mg
		S is 1 ml
Means = Extremes	0.2A = 24	$\dfrac{24 \text{ mg}}{0.2 \text{ mg}} \times 1 \text{ ml} = \mathbf{A} \text{ ml}$
0.2A = 24	A = 120	
A = 120 ml/hr	You will run the pump at	A = 120 ml
You will run the pump at **120 ml/hr**	**120 ml/hr**	You will run the pump at **120 ml/hr**

5. Doctor's order reads *dobutamine 5 mcg/kg/min IV for 6 hours.* The bag of dobutamine has a concentration of **1 mg/ml.** The patient weighs **55 kg.** At what flow rate will you run the pump?

    Calculate the amount of drug/minute.
    Multiply the dose by the patient's weight.
    5 mcg × 55 kg = 275 mcg

The patient will get 275 mcg/minute.

Convert mcg/min to mg/min.

275 mcg = 0.275 mg/min

Convert minutes to mcg/min to mg/hour.

0.275 mcg/min = 0.275 × 60 = 16.5 mg/hr

Ratio and Proportion: Means = Extremes	**Ratio and Proportion: Cross Multiplication of Fractions**	**Formula**
Known ratio 1 mg : 1 ml Unknown ratio 16.5 mg : A ml	Known ratio $\dfrac{1\ mg}{1\ ml}$	$\dfrac{\text{Dose \textbf{D}esired}}{\text{Dose on \textbf{H}and}} \times \textbf{S}\text{tock}$
16.5 mg : A ml : 1 mg : 1 ml	Unknown ratio $\dfrac{16.5\ mg}{A\ ml}$	$= \textbf{A}\text{mount}$
Means = 1 × A = A Extremes = 16.5 × 1 = 16.5	$\dfrac{16.5\ mg}{A\ ml} \; \nwarrow \nearrow \; \dfrac{1\ mg}{1\ ml}$ $\swarrow \searrow$	$\dfrac{\textbf{D}}{\textbf{H}} \times \textbf{S} = \textbf{A}$ **D** is 16.5 mg **H** is 1 mg **S** is 1 ml
Means = Extremes A = 16.5 You will run the pump at **16.5 ml/hr**	A = 16.5 You will run the pump at **16.5 ml/hr**	$\dfrac{16.5\ mg}{1\ mg} \times 1\ ml = \textbf{A}\ ml$ A = 16.5 ml You will run the pump at **16.5 ml/hr**

CHAPTER 14

MIXING TWO PREPARATIONS OF INSULIN IN ONE SYRINGE

On the following insulin syringes, mark the amount of regular insulin and the total amount of insulin prescribed in the following doctor's orders.

1. *Regular insulin 17 u and NPH insulin 28 u.*

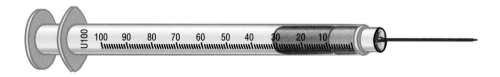

2. *Regular insulin 9 u and NPH insulin 22 u.*

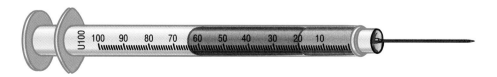

3. *Regular insulin 20 u and NPH insulin 44 u.*

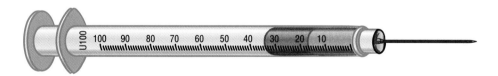

4. *Regular insulin 12 u and NPH insulin 37 u.*

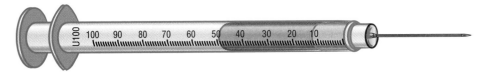

5. *Regular insulin 5 u and NPH insulin 16 u.*

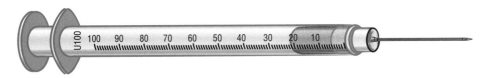

Titrated Insulin

The doctor's order reads
Regular insulin sc by glucometer TID AC and HS
     blood sugar   0–9.9 no insulin
                 10.0–14.9 give 6 units
                 15.0–19.9 give 8 units
                 20.0–24.9 give 10 units

Using the above doctor's order, how much insulin will you give in the following situations?

1. At 0730 hrs your patient's blood sugar is 8.4.

     no insulin

2. At 1130 hrs your patient's blood sugar is 17.0.

     8 units

3. At 1730 hrs your patient's blood sugar is 13.7.

     6 units

4. At 2200 hrs your patient's blood sugar is 12.5.

     6 units

CHAPTER 15

The label on the vial of heparin reads **heparin 10 000 u/ml.** How much heparin will you draw up for each of the following doctor's orders?

1. *Heparin 5 000 u sc bid*

Ratio and Proportion:
Means = Extremes

Known ratio   10 000 u : 1 ml
Unknown ratio   5 000 u : A ml

5 000 u : A ml : 10 000 u : 1 ml

Means = 10 000 × A
    = 10 000A
Extremes = 5 000 × 1 = 5 000

10 000A = 5 000

A = 0.5 ml

Ratio and Proportion:
Cross Multiplication of
Fractions

Known ratio $\dfrac{10\,000\ u}{1\ ml}$

Unknown ratio $\dfrac{5\,000}{A\ ml}$

$\dfrac{5\,000}{A\ ml}\ \nwarrow\ \nearrow\ \dfrac{10\,000\ u}{1\ ml}$
$\qquad\ \swarrow\ \searrow$

10 000A = 5 000

A = 0.5 ml

Formula

$\dfrac{\text{Dose \textbf{D}esired}}{\text{Dose on \textbf{H}and}} \times \textbf{S}\text{tock}$

    = **A**mount

$\dfrac{\textbf{D}}{\textbf{H}} \times \textbf{S} = \textbf{A}$

D is 5 000 u
H is 10 000 u
S is 1 ml

$\dfrac{5\,000\ u}{10\,000\ u} \times 1\ ml = \textbf{A}\ ml$

A = 0.5 ml

2. *Heparin 2 500 u sc qid*

Ratio and Proportion: Means = Extremes

Known ratio   10 000 u : 1 ml
Unknown ratio 2 500 u : A ml

2 500 u : A ml : 10 000 u : 1 ml

Means = 10 000 × A
    = 10 000A
Extremes = 2 500 × 1 = 2 500

10 000A = 2 500

A = 0.25 ml

Ratio and Proportion: Cross Multiplication of Fractions

Known Ratio $\dfrac{10\ 000\ u}{1\ ml}$

Unknown Ratio $\dfrac{2\ 500}{A\ ml}$

$\dfrac{2\ 500\ u}{A\ ml} \nwarrow \nearrow \dfrac{10\ 000\ u}{1\ ml}$

10 000 A = 2 500

A = 0.25 ml

Formula

$\dfrac{Dose\ \mathbf{D}esired}{Dose\ on\ \mathbf{H}and} \times \mathbf{S}tock$
   $= \mathbf{A}mount$

$\dfrac{\mathbf{D}}{\mathbf{H}} \times \mathbf{S} = \mathbf{A}$

D is 2 500 u
H is 10 000 u
S is 1 ml

$\dfrac{2\ 500\ u}{10\ 000\ u} \times 1\ ml = \mathbf{A}\ ml$

A = 0.25 ml

3. *Heparin 4 000 u sc bid*

Ratio and Proportion: Means = Extremes

Known ratio   10 000 u : 1 ml
Unknown ratio 4 000 u : A ml

4 000 u : A ml : 10 000 u : 1 ml

Means = 10 000 × A
    = 10 000 A
Extremes = 4 000 × 1
    = 4 000

10 000A = 4 000
A = 0.4 ml

Ratio and Proportion: Cross Multiplication of Fractions

Known ratio $\dfrac{10\ 000\ u}{1\ ml}$

Unknown ratio $\dfrac{4\ 000}{A\ ml}$

$\dfrac{4\ 000}{A\ ml} \nwarrow \nearrow \dfrac{10\ 000\ u}{1\ ml}$

10 000A = 4 000

A = 0.4 ml

Formula

$\dfrac{Dose\ \mathbf{D}esired}{Dose\ on\ \mathbf{H}and} \times \mathbf{S}tock$
   $= \mathbf{A}mount$

$\dfrac{\mathbf{D}}{\mathbf{H}} \times \mathbf{S} = \mathbf{A}$

D is 4 000 u
H is 10 000 u
S is 1 ml

$\dfrac{4\ 000\ u}{10\ 000\ u} \times 1\ ml = \mathbf{A}\ ml$

A = 0.4 ml

4. *Heparin 5 500 u sc bid*

Ratio and Proportion: Means = Extremes

Known ratio   10 000 u : 1 ml
Unknown ratio 5 500 u : A ml

5 500 u : A ml : 10 000 u : 1 ml

Means = 10 000 × A
    = 10 000A
Extremes = 5 500 × 1 = 5 500

10 000A = 5 500

A = 0.55 ml

Ratio and Proportion: Cross Multiplication of Fractions

Known ratio $\dfrac{10\ 000\ u}{1\ ml}$

Unknown ratio $\dfrac{5\ 500}{A\ ml}$

$\dfrac{5\ 00}{A\ ml} \nwarrow \nearrow \dfrac{10\ 000\ u}{1\ ml}$

10 000A = 5 500

A = 0.55 ml

Formula

$\dfrac{Dose\ \mathbf{D}esired}{Dose\ on\ \mathbf{H}and} \times \mathbf{S}tock$
   $= \mathbf{A}mount$

$\dfrac{\mathbf{D}}{\mathbf{H}} \times \mathbf{S} = \mathbf{A}$

D is 5 500 u
H is 10 000 u
S is 1 ml

$\dfrac{5\ 500\ u}{10\ 000\ u} \times 1\ ml = \mathbf{A}\ ml$

A = 0.55 ml

Calculate the IV flow rate for each of the following heparin orders. All orders will use the standard IV concentration of heparin of 25 000 u/250 ml NS or 100 u/ml.

1. Doctor's order reads *heparin IV 1 200 u/hr.*

Ratio and Proportion: Means = Extremes

Known ratio   100 u : 1 ml
Unknown ratio   1 200 : A ml

1 200 u : A ml : 100 u : 1 ml

Means = 100 × A = 100 A
Extremes = 1 200 × 1 = 1 200

Means = Extremes
100A = 1 200
A = 12

You will run the pump at **12 ml/hr.**

Ratio and Proportion: Cross Multiplication of Fractions

Known ratio $\dfrac{100\ u}{1\ ml}$

Unknown ratio $\dfrac{1\ 200\ u}{A\ ml}$

$\dfrac{1\ 200\ u}{A\ ml}$ ↖ ↗ $\dfrac{100\ u}{1\ ml}$ ↙ ↘

100A = 1200
A = 12

You will run the pump at **12 ml/hr.**

Formula

$\dfrac{\text{Dose } \mathbf{D}\text{esired}}{\text{Dose on } \mathbf{H}\text{and}} \times \mathbf{S}\text{tock}$

$= \mathbf{A}\text{mount}$

$\dfrac{\mathbf{D}}{\mathbf{H}} \times \mathbf{S} = \mathbf{A}$

D is 1 200 u
H is 100 u
S is 1 ml

$\dfrac{1\ 200}{100\ u} \times 1\ ml = \mathbf{A}\ ml$

A = 12 ml

You will run the pump at **12 ml/hr.**

2. Doctor's order *heparin IV 1 000 u/hr.*

Ratio and Proportion: Means = Extremes

Known ratio   100 u : 1 ml
Unknown ratio   1 000 : A ml

1 000 u : A ml : 100 u : 1 ml

Means = 100 × A = 100 A
Extremes = 1 000 × 1 = 1 200

Means = Extremes
100A = 1 000
A = 10

You will run the pump at **10 ml/hr.**

Ratio and Proportion: Cross Multiplication of Fractions

Known ratio $\dfrac{100\ u}{1\ ml}$

Unknown ratio $\dfrac{1\ 000\ u}{A\ ml}$

$\dfrac{1\ 000\ u}{A\ ml}$ ↖ ↗ $\dfrac{100\ u}{1\ ml}$ ↙ ↘

100A = 1 000
A = 10

You will run the pump at **10 ml/hr.**

Formula

$\dfrac{\text{Dose } \mathbf{D}\text{esired}}{\text{Dose on } \mathbf{H}\text{and}} \times \mathbf{S}\text{tock}$

$= \mathbf{A}\text{mount}$

$\dfrac{\mathbf{D}}{\mathbf{H}} \times \mathbf{S} = \mathbf{A}$

D is 1 000 u
H is 100 u
S is 1 ml

$\dfrac{1\ 000}{100\ u} \times 1\ ml = \mathbf{A}\ ml$

A = 10 ml

You will run the pump at **10 ml/hr.**

3. Doctor's order reads *heparin IV 19u/kg/hr.* Patient's weight is 88 kg.

Calculate the amount of drug/hour. Multiply the dose by the patient's weight.
19 u × 88 = 1 672 u/hr

The patient will get 1 672 u/hr.

Ratio and Proportion: Means = Extremes

Known ratio   100 u : 1 ml
Unknown ratio   1 672 : A ml

1 672 u : A ml : 100 u : 1 ml

Means = 100 × A = 100A
Extremes = 1 672 × 1 = 1 672

Means = Extremes
100A = 1 672
A = 16.72
Convert to a whole
number = 17

You will run the pump at
17 ml/hr.

Ratio and Proportion: Cross Multiplication of Fractions

Known ratio $\dfrac{100\ u}{1\ ml}$

Unknown ratio $\dfrac{1\ 672\ u}{A\ ml}$

$\dfrac{1\ 672\ u}{A\ ml}$ ↖ ↗ $\dfrac{100\ u}{1\ ml}$
  ↙ ↘

100A = 1 672
A = 16.72

Convert to a whole
number = 17

You will run the pump at
17 ml/hr.

Formula

$\dfrac{\text{Dose } \textbf{D}\text{esired}}{\text{Dose on } \textbf{H}\text{and}} \times \textbf{S}\text{tock}$
    $= \textbf{A}\text{mount}$

$\dfrac{\textbf{D}}{\textbf{H}} \times \textbf{S} = \textbf{A}$

D is 1 672 u
H is 100 u
S is 1 ml

$\dfrac{1\ 672}{100\ u} \times 1\ ml = \textbf{A}\ ml$

A = 16.72 ml
Convert to a whole
number = 17

You will run the pump at
17 ml/hr.

4. Doctor's order reads *heparin IV 17 u/kg/hr.* Patient's weight is 55 kg.

   Calculate the amount of drug/hour. Multiply the dose by the patient's weight.
   17 u × 55 = 935 u/hr

   The patient will get 935 u/hr.

Ratio and Proportion: Means = Extremes

Known ratio   100 u : 1 ml
Unknown ratio   935 : A ml

1 672 u : A ml : 100 u : 1 ml

Means = 100 × A = 100A
Extremes = 935 × 1 = 935

Means = Extremes
100A = 935
A = 9.35
Convert to a whole
number = 9

You will run the pump at
9 ml/hr

Ratio and Proportion: Cross Multiplication of Fractions

Known ratio $\dfrac{100\ u}{1\ ml}$

Unknown ratio $\dfrac{935\ u}{A\ ml}$

$\dfrac{935\ u}{A\ ml}$ ↖ ↗ $\dfrac{100\ u}{1\ ml}$
  ↙ ↘

100A = 935
A = 9.35

Convert to a whole
number = 9

You will run the pump at
9 ml/hr.

Formula

$\dfrac{\text{Dose } \textbf{D}\text{esired}}{\text{Dose on } \textbf{H}\text{and}} \times \textbf{S}\text{tock}$
    $= \textbf{A}\text{mount}$

$\dfrac{\textbf{D}}{\textbf{H}} \times \textbf{S} = \textbf{A}$

D is 935 u
H is 100 u
S is 1 ml

$\dfrac{935\ u}{100\ u} \times 1\ ml = \textbf{A}\ ml$

A = 9.35 ml
Convert to a whole
number = 9

You will run the pump at
9 ml/hr.

5. Doctor's order reads *heparin IV 22 u/kg/hr.* Patient's weight is 73 kg.

Calculate the amount of drug/hour. Multiply the dose by the patient's weight. 22 u × 73 = 1 606 u/hr

The patient will get 1 606 u/hr.

Ratio and Proportion: Means = Extremes	Ratio and Proportion: Cross Multiplication of Fractions	Formula

Known ratio   100 u : 1 ml
Unknown ratio 1 606 : A ml
 	
1 606 u : A ml : 100 u : 1 ml
 	
Means = 100 × A = 100A
Extremes = 1 606 × 1 = 1 606
 	
Means = Extremes
100A = 1 606
A = 16.06
Convert to a whole
  number = 16
 	
You will run the pump at
16 ml/hr.
	Known ratio $\dfrac{100\ u}{1\ ml}$
	
	Unknown ratio $\dfrac{1\ 606\ u}{A\ ml}$
	
	$\dfrac{1\ 606\ u}{A\ ml}\ \nwarrow\nearrow\ \dfrac{100\ u}{1\ ml}\ \swarrow\searrow$
	
	100A = 1 606
	A = 16.06
	
	Convert to a whole
	  number = 16
	
	You will run the pump at
	16 ml/hr.
		$\dfrac{\text{Dose } \mathbf{D}\text{esired}}{\text{Dose on } \mathbf{H}\text{and}} \times \mathbf{S}\text{tock}$
		$\quad = \mathbf{A}\text{mount}$
		
		$\dfrac{\mathbf{D}}{\mathbf{H}} \times \mathbf{S} = \mathbf{A}$
		
		D is 1 606 u
		H is 100 u
		S is 1 ml
		
		$\dfrac{1\ 606\ u}{100\ u} \times 1\ ml = \mathbf{A}\ ml$
		
		A = 16.06 ml
		
		Convert to a whole
		  number = 16
		
		You will run the pump at
		16 ml/hr.

CHAPTER 16

MEDICATIONS ORDERED IN DOSE/KG

1. Helena is a 6-month-old girl who weighs 5 kg. The doctor's order reads *gentamycin 1 mg/kg IV q12h.* The label on the vial reads **gentamycin 10 mg/ml.** How much gentamycin should you draw up?

Dose of drug (mg/kg) × weight (kg) = mg of drug

1 mg/kg × 5 kg = **5 mg of gentamycin**

Ratio and Proportion: Means = Extremes	Ratio and Proportion: Cross Multiplication of Fractions	Formula
The known ratio is 10 mg : 1 ml The unknown ratio is 5 mg : A ml $\qquad\downarrow$-means-$\downarrow$ $\quad$ 5:A $\quad=\quad$ 10:1 $\qquad\uparrow$---extremes----$\uparrow$ Means = Extremes 10A = 5 A = **0.5 ml**	Known ratio is 10 mg in 1 ml $\dfrac{10}{1}$ Unknown ratio is 5 mg in A ml $\dfrac{5}{A}$ $\dfrac{5\ mg}{A\ ml}\ \nwarrow\nearrow\ \dfrac{10\ mg}{1\ ml}\ \swarrow\searrow$ 10A = 5 A = **0.5 ml**	$\dfrac{\text{Dose } \mathbf{D}\text{esired (mg)}}{\text{Dose on } \mathbf{H}\text{and (mg)}}$ $\quad \times \mathbf{S}\text{tock (ml)} = \mathbf{A}\text{mount}$ or $\dfrac{\mathbf{D}}{\mathbf{H}} \times \mathbf{S} = \mathbf{A}$ Dose **D**esired is 5 mg Dose on **H**and is 10 mg **S**tock is 1 ml $\dfrac{5\ mg}{10\ mg} \times 1\ ml = \mathbf{A}$ A = **0.5 ml** You will draw up **0.5 ml** of gentamycin.

2. Ramon is a 17-month-old boy who weighs 6.3 kg. The doctor's order reads *ondansetron 0.1 mg/kg IV q8h PRN for nausea and vomiting*. The label on the vial reads **ondansetron 2 mg/ml.** How much ondansetron should you draw up?

Dose of drug (mg/kg) $\times$ weight (kg) = mg of drug

0.1 mg/kg $\times$ 6.3 kg = 0.63 mg of ondansetron

Ratio and Proportion: Means = Extremes	**Ratio and Proportion: Cross Multiplication of Fractions**	**Formula**
The known ratio is 2 mg : 1 ml The unknown ratio is 0.63 mg : A ml	Known ratio is 2 mg in 1 ml $\frac{2}{1}$	$\dfrac{\text{Dose \textbf{D}esired (mg)}}{\text{Dose on \textbf{H}and (mg)}}$ $\times$ **S**tock (ml) = **A**mount
$\downarrow$-means-$\downarrow$ 0.63:A = 2:1 $\uparrow$----extremes----$\uparrow$	Unknown ratio is 0.63 mg in A ml $\frac{0.63}{A}$	or $\dfrac{\textbf{D}}{\textbf{H}} \times \textbf{S} = \textbf{A}$
Means = Extremes	$\dfrac{0.63 \text{ mg}}{A \text{ ml}} \nwarrow \nearrow \dfrac{2 \text{ mg}}{1 \text{ ml}}$	Dose **D**esired is 0.63 mg Dose on **H**and is 2 mg **S**tock is 1 ml
2A = 0.63	2A = 0.63	$\dfrac{0.63 \text{ mg}}{2 \text{ mg}} \times 1 \text{ ml} = \textbf{A}$
A = **0.3 ml**	A = **0.3 ml**	A = **0.3 ml** You will draw up **0.3 ml** of ondansetron.

3. Natasha is a 3-year-old girl who weighs 14.7 kg. The doctor's order reads *Cefizox (ceftizoxime) 50 mg/kg IV Q8H.* The label on the vial reads **Cefizox 1 gram.** The dilution instructions state that you should add 3 ml of normal saline to get a concentration of 270 mg/ml. How much Cefizox should you draw up?

Dose of drug (mg/kg) $\times$ weight (kg) = mg of drug

50 mg/kg $\times$ 14.7 = 735 mg of Cefizox

Ratio and Proportion: Means = Extremes	**Ratio and Proportion: Cross Multiplication of Fractions**	**Formula**
The known ratio is 270 mg : 1 ml The unknown ratio is 735 mg : A ml	Known ratio is 270 mg in 1 ml $\frac{270}{1}$	$\dfrac{\text{Dose \textbf{D}esired (mg)}}{\text{Dose on \textbf{H}and (mg)}}$ $\times$ **S**tock (ml) = **A**mount
$\downarrow$-means-$\downarrow$ 735:A = 270:1 $\uparrow$----extremes-----$\uparrow$	Unknown ratio is 735 mg in A ml $\frac{735}{A}$	or $\dfrac{\textbf{D}}{\textbf{H}} \times \textbf{S} = \textbf{A}$
Means = Extremes	$\dfrac{735 \text{ mg}}{A \text{ ml}} \nwarrow \nearrow \dfrac{270 \text{ mg}}{1 \text{ ml}}$	Dose **D**esired is 735 mg Dose on **H**and is 270 mg **S**tock is 1 ml
270A = 735	270A = 735	$\dfrac{735 \text{ mg}}{270 \text{ mg}} \times 1 \text{ ml} = \textbf{A}$
A = **2.7 ml**	A = **2.7 ml**	A = **2.7 ml** You will draw up **2.7 ml** of Cefizox.

4. MacKenzie is a 6-year-old girl who weighs 21.4 kg. The doctor's order reads *Ceclor (cefaclor)10 mg/kg po q8h.* The label on the bottle reads **Ceclor 375 mg/5 ml.** How much Ceclor should you administer?

Dose of drug (mg/kg) × weight (kg) = mg of Ceclor

10 mg/kg × 21.4 kg = 214 mg of Ceclor

Ratio and Proportion: Means = Extremes	**Ratio and Proportion: Cross Multiplication of Fractions**	**Formula**
The known ratio is 375 mg : 5 ml The unknown ratio is 214 mg : A ml	Known ratio is 375 mg in 5 ml $\dfrac{375}{5}$	$\dfrac{\text{Dose } \textbf{D}\text{esired (mg)}}{\text{Dose on } \textbf{H}\text{and (mg)}}$ × **S**tock (ml) = **A**mount
↓-means-↓ 214 : A = 375 : 5 ↑----extremes-----↑	Unknown ratio is 214 mg in A ml $\dfrac{214}{A}$	or $\dfrac{\textbf{D}}{\textbf{H}} \times \textbf{S} = \textbf{A}$
Means = Extremes	$\dfrac{214 \text{ mg}}{A \text{ ml}} \nwarrow \nearrow \dfrac{375 \text{ mg}}{5 \text{ ml}}$ $\swarrow \searrow$	Dose **D**esired is 214 mg Dose on **H**and is 375 mg **S**tock is 5 ml
375A = 1 070	375A = 1 070	$\dfrac{214 \text{ mg}}{375 \text{ mg}} \times 5 \text{ ml} = \textbf{A}$
A = **2.9 ml**	A = **2.9 ml**	A = **2.9 ml**
		You will administer **2.9 ml** of Ceclor.

5. Armand is a 10-year-old boy who weighs 35 kg. The doctor's order reads *Flagyl (metronidazole) 10 mg/kg IV.* Flagyl comes premixed in a 100-ml bag with a strength of 500 mg/100 ml. How much of the Flagyl will you administer?

Dose of drug (mg/kg) × weight (kg) = mg of drug

10 mg/kg × 35 kg = 350 mg of Flagyl

Ratio and Proportion: Means = Extremes	**Ratio and Proportion: Cross Multiplication of Fractions**	**Formula**
The known ratio is 500 mg : 100 ml The unknown ratio is 350 mg : A ml	Known ratio is 500 mg in 100 ml $\dfrac{500}{100}$	$\dfrac{\text{Dose } \textbf{D}\text{esired (mg)}}{\text{Dose on } \textbf{H}\text{and (mg)}}$ × **S**tock (ml) = **A**mount
↓-means-↓ 350 : A = 500 : 100 ↑-----extremes------↑	Unknown ratio is 350 mg in A ml $\dfrac{350}{A}$	or $\dfrac{\textbf{D}}{\textbf{H}} \times \textbf{S} = \textbf{A}$
Means = Extremes	$\dfrac{350 \text{ mg}}{A \text{ ml}} \nwarrow \nearrow \dfrac{500 \text{ mg}}{100 \text{ ml}}$ $\swarrow \searrow$	Dose **D**esired is 350 mg Dose on **H**and is 500 mg **S**tock is 100 ml
500A = 35 000	500A = 35 000	$\dfrac{350 \text{ mg}}{500 \text{ mg}} \times 100 \text{ ml} = \textbf{A}$
A = **70 ml**	A = **70 ml**	A = **70 ml**
		You will administer **70 ml** of Flagyl.

CALCULATION OF BODY SURFACE AREA (BSA)

1. A 22-month-old girl is 82 cm tall and weighs 13 kg.

    $$BSA \ (m^2) = \sqrt{\frac{weight \ (kg) \times height \ (cm)}{3\ 600}}$$

    $$BSA \ (m^2) = \sqrt{\frac{13 \ kg \times 82 \ cm}{3\ 600}}$$

    $$BSA = \textbf{0.54 m}^2$$

2. A 2-month-old boy is 57 cm long and weighs 4.6 kg.

    $$BSA \ (m^2) = \sqrt{\frac{weight \ (kg) \times height \ (cm)}{3\ 600}}$$

    $$BSA \ (m^2) = \sqrt{\frac{4.6 \ kg \times 57 \ cm}{3\ 600}}$$

    $$BSA = \textbf{0.27 m}^2$$

3. A 5-year-old girl is 103 cm tall and weighs 16 kg.

    $$BSA \ (m^2) = \sqrt{\frac{weight \ (kg) \times height \ (cm)}{3\ 600}}$$

    $$BSA \ (m^2) = \sqrt{\frac{16 \ kg \times 103 \ cm}{3\ 600}}$$

    $$BSA = \textbf{0.68 m}^2$$

4. A 10-year-old boy is 144 cm tall and weighs 42 kg.

    $$BSA \ (m^2) = \sqrt{\frac{weight \ (kg) \times height \ (cm)}{3\ 600}}$$

    $$BSA \ (m^2) = \sqrt{\frac{42 \ kg \times 144 \ cm}{3\ 600}}$$

    $$BSA = \textbf{1.3 m}^2$$

5. A 15-year-old boy us 180 cm tall and weighs 75 kg.

    $$BSA \ (m^2) = \sqrt{\frac{weight \ (kg) \times height \ (cm)}{3\ 600}}$$

    $$BSA \ (m^2) = \sqrt{\frac{75 \ kg \times 180 \ cm}{3\ 600}}$$

    $$BSA = \textbf{1.93 m}^2$$

MEDICATIONS ORDERED IN DOSE/m²

1. Brian is a 16-year-old boy with a diagnosis of Hodgkin's disease. He is 158 cm tall and weighs 43 kg. The doctor's order reads *Blenoxane (bleomycin) 15 u/m² IV twice weekly*. The label on the vial reads **Blenoxane 15 u.** The directions on the vial state that the drug should be reconstituted with 10 ml of normal saline. How much Blenoxane will you draw up?

Calculation of BSA

$$BSA \ (m^2) = \sqrt{\frac{weight \ (kg) \times height \ (cm)}{3\ 600}}$$

$$BSA \ (m^2) = \sqrt{\frac{43 \ kg \times 158 \ cm}{3\ 600}}$$

$$= 1.37 \ m^2$$

Calculation of dose of drug

Dose of drug mg/u $\times$ BSA (m^2) = u of drug

15 mg/ m^2 $\times$ 1.37 m^2 = 20.6 u of Blenoxane

Calculation of amount of drug to give

Ratio and Proportion: **Means = Extremes**	**Ratio and Proportion:** **Cross Multiplication of Fractions**	**Formula**
The known ratio is 15 u : 10 ml The unknown ratio is 20.6 u : A ml	Known ratio is 15 u in $\frac{15}{10}$ 10 ml	$\dfrac{Dose \ \mathbf{D}esired \ (mg)}{Dose \ on \ \mathbf{H}and \ (mg)}$ $\times \ \mathbf{S}tock \ (ml) = \mathbf{A}mount$
↓-means-↓ 20.6:A = 15:10 ↑----extremes-----↑	Unknown ratio is 20.6 u in A ml $\frac{20.6}{A}$	or $\dfrac{\mathbf{D}}{\mathbf{H}} \times \mathbf{S} = \mathbf{A}$
Means = Extremes	$\dfrac{20.6 \ u}{A \ ml} \nwarrow \nearrow \dfrac{15u}{10 \ ml}$	Dose **D**esired is 20.6 u Dose on **H**and is 15 u **S**tock is 10 ml
15A = 206	15A = 206	$\dfrac{20.6 \ mg}{15 \ mg} \times 10 \ ml = \mathbf{A}$
A = **13.7 ml**	A = **13.7 ml**	A = **13.7 ml** Blenoxane.

2. Susan is a 3-year-old girl with a diagnosis of acute lymphocytic leukemia. She is 93 cm tall and weighs 12 kg. The doctor's order reads *Myleran (busulfan) 1.8 mg/m² po daily.* The label on the bottle of tablets reads **Myleran 2 mg tablets.** The package material states that the tablets may be cut in half. How many tablets of Myleran will you administer?

Calculation of BSA

$$BSA \ (m^2) = \sqrt{\frac{weight \ (kg) \times height \ (cm)}{3\ 600}}$$

$$BSA \ (m^2) = \sqrt{\frac{12 \ kg \times 93 \ cm}{3\ 600}}$$

$$= 0.56 \ m^2$$

Calculation of dose of drug

Dose of drug mg/kg $\times$ BSA (m^2) = mg of drug

1.8 mg/m^2 $\times$ 0.56 m^2 = 1 mg of Myleran

Ratio and Proportion: Means = Extremes

The known ratio is
2 mg : 1 tablet
The unknown ratio is
1 mg : A tablets

↓-means-↓
1 : A   =   2 : 1
↑--extremes---↑

Means = Extremes

2A = 1

A = **0.5 tablets**

Ratio and Proportion: Cross Multiplication of Fractions

Known ratio is 2 mg in

1 tablet $\dfrac{2}{1}$

Unknown ratio is 1 mg in

A tablets $\dfrac{1}{A}$

$\dfrac{1\ mg}{A\ tablets}$ ↖ ↗ $\dfrac{2\ mg}{1\ tablet}$

2A = 1

A = **0.5 tablets**

Formula

$\dfrac{\text{Dose } \textbf{D}\text{esired (mg)}}{\text{Dose on } \textbf{H}\text{and (mg)}}$

$\times\ \textbf{S}\text{tock (ml)} = \textbf{A}\text{mount}$

or $\dfrac{\textbf{D}}{\textbf{H}} \times \textbf{S} = \textbf{A}$

Dose **D**esired is 1 mg
Dose on **H**and is 2 mg
Stock is 1 tablet

$\dfrac{1\ mg}{2\ mg} \times 1\ \text{tablet} = \textbf{A}$

A = **0.5 ml**

You will give $^1/_2$ **tablet** of Myleran.

3. Sean is a 2-year-old boy with a diagnosis of Letterer-Siwe disease. He is 88 cm tall and weighs 13.2 kg. His doctor's orders read *vinblastine IV once weekly according to the following schedule for 5 weeks.*

June 7	*2.5 mg/m²*
June 14	*3.75 mg/m²*
June 21	*5 mg/m²*
June 28	*6.25 mg/m²*
July 5	*7.5 mg/m²*

The label on the vial reads **vinblastine 1 mg/ml.** How much vinblastine will you draw up on each date?

$$\text{BSA (m}^2) = \sqrt{\dfrac{\text{weight (kg)} \times \text{height (cm)}}{3\ 600}}$$

$$\text{BSA (m}^2) = \sqrt{\dfrac{13.2\ \text{kg} \times 88\ \text{cm}}{3\ 600}}$$

$$= \textbf{0.57 m}^2$$

June 7   2.5 mg/m²

Calculation of dose of drug

Dose of drug mg/m² × BSA (m²) = mg of drug

2.5 mg/m² × 0.57 m² = 1.4 mg vinblastine

Strength of drug is 1 mg/ml so you will administer **1.4 ml** of vinblastine.

June 14   3.75 mg/m²

Calculation of dose of drug

Dose of drug mg/kg × BSA (m²) = mg of drug

3.75 mg/m² × 0.57 m² = 2.1 mg of vinblastine

Strength of drug is 1 mg/ml so you will administer **2.1 ml** of vinblastine.

June 21   5 mg/m²

Calculation of dose of drug

Dose of drug mg/kg × BSA (m²) = mg of drug

5 mg/m² × 0.57 m² = 2.9 mg vinblastine

Strength of drug is 1 mg/ml so you will administer **2.9 ml** of vinblastine.

June 28   6.25 mg/m²

Calculation of dose of drug

Dose of drug mg/kg × BSA (m²) = mg of drug

6.25 mg/m² × 0.57 m² = 3.6 mg vinblastine

Strength of drug is 1 mg/ml so you will administer **3.6 ml** of vinblastine.

July 5   7.5 mg/m²

Calculation of dose of drug

Dose of drug mg/kg × BSA (m²) = mg of drug

7.5 mg/m² × 0.57 m² = 4.3 mg vinblastine

Strength of drug is 1 mg/ml so you will administer **4.3 ml** of vinblastine.

CALCULATION OF SAFE DOSAGE

1. Henry is 3 years old and has been admitted with croup. The doctor's order reads *acetaminophen suppository 80 mg pr Q4H PRN*. The maximum dose in 24 hours is 720 mg. If the medication is given as often as possible, will the maximum dose be exceeded?

Calculate the number of doses of drug in 24 hours.

$$\frac{24 \text{ hours}}{\text{frequency (hours)}} = \text{number of doses of drug}$$

$$\frac{24 \text{ hours}}{4 \text{ hours}} = 6 \text{ doses}$$

Calculate the total dose of drug to be given in 24 hours.

Single dose of drug × the number of doses in 24 hours = total dose of drug

80 mg × 6 = 480 mg

Compare the total dose of the drug to be given to the maximum safe dose.

Maximum safe dose is 720 mg

480 mg is less than 720, so **the dose is safe to give.**

2. Elena is a 10-year-old girl who weighs 27.5 kg. The doctor's order reads *Pepcid (famotidine) 0.5 mg/kg IV Q8H*. The maximum daily dose is 40 mg/day. Is this dose within the safe range?

   Calculate the dose of the medication (if necessary).

   Dose of drug mg/kg × weight (kg) = mg of drug

   0.5 mg/kg × 27.5 kg = 13.8 mg of Pepcid

   Calculate the number of doses of drug in 24 hours.

   $$\frac{24 \text{ hours}}{\text{frequency (hours)}} = \text{number of doses of drug}$$

   $$\frac{24 \text{ hours}}{8 \text{ hours}} = 3$$

   Calculate the total dose of drug to be given in 24 hours.

   Single dose of drug × the number of doses in 24 hours = total dose of drug

   13.8 mg × 3 = 41.4 mg

   Compare the total dose of the drug to be given to the maximum safe dose.

   Maximum safe dose is 40 mg

   41.4 is more than 40 mg, so **the dose should be questioned.**

3. Randi is a 5-year-old girl who weighs 18.5 kg. The doctor's order reads *Keflex cephalexin) suspension 250 mg po qid*. The safe dosage range for this drug is 25–100 mg/kg/day. Is this dose within the safe range?

   Calculate the safe minimum daily dose.

   Minimum safe dose of drug (mg/kg) × weight (kg) = mg of drug

   25 mg/kg × 18.5 kg = 462.5 mg Keflex

   Calculate the safe maximum daily dose.

   Maximum safe dose of drug (mg/kg) × weight (kg) = mg of drug

   100 mg/kg × 18.5 kg = 1 850 mg

   Calculate the number of doses of drug in 24 hours.

   Drug is ordered 4 times/day

   Calculate the total dose of drug to be given in 24 hours.

   Single dose of drug × the number of doses in 24 hours = total dose of drug

   250 mg × 4 = 1 000 mg

   Compare the total dose of the drug to be given to the minimum and maximum safe doses.

   Minimum safe dose is 462.5 mg

   Maximum safe dose is 1 850 mg

Total amount ordered is 1 000 mg

This amount falls between the minimum and maximum safe doses, so **it is safe to give.**

4. Jared is a 7-year-old boy who weighs 22 kg. The doctor's order reads *phenobarbital 40 mg IV QHS.* The safe dosage range for this drug is 1–3 mg/kg/day. Is this dose within the safe range?

Calculate the safe minimum daily dose.

Minimum safe dose of drug (mg/kg) × weight (kg) = mg of drug

1 mg/kg × 22 kg = 22 mg

Calculate the safe maximum daily dose.

Maximum safe dose of drug (mg/kg) × weight (kg) = mg of drug

3 mg/kg × 22 kg = 66 mg

Calculate the number of doses of drug in 24 hours.

Drug is ordered once per day

Calculate the total dose of drug to be given in 24 hours.

Total dose in 24 hours is 40 mg

Compare the total dose of the drug to be given to the minimum and maximum safe doses.

Minimum safe dose is 22 mg

Maximum safe dose is 66 mg

Total amount ordered is 40 mg

This amount falls between the minimum and maximum safe doses, so **it is safe to give.**

5. Maria is a 5-year-old girl who weighs 17 kg. The doctor's order reads *penicillin 150 000 u IV Q4H.* The safe dosage range for this drug is 25 000–300 000 u/kg/day. Is this dose within the safe range?

Calculate the safe minimum daily dose.

Minimum safe dose of drug (u/kg) × weight (kg) = u of drug

25 000 u/kg × 17 kg = 425 000 u

Calculate the safe maximum daily dose.

Maximum safe dose of drug (u/kg) × weight (kg) = u of drug

300 000 u/kg × 17 kg = 5 100 000 u

Calculate the number of doses of drug in 24 hours.

$$\frac{24 \text{ hours}}{\text{frequency (hours)}} = \text{number of doses of drug}$$

$$\frac{24 \text{ hours}}{4 \text{ hours}} = 6$$

Calculate the total dose of drug to be given in 24 hours.

Single dose of drug × the number of doses in 24 hours = total dose of drug

150 000 u × 6 = 900 000 u

Compare the total dose of the drug to be given to the minimum and maximum safe doses.

Minimum safe dose is 425 000 u

Maximum safe dose is 5 100 000 u

Total amount ordered is 900 000 u

This amount falls between the minimum and maximum safe doses, so **it is safe to give.**

CALCULATION OF FLUID REQUIREMENTS FOR CHILDREN

Identify the appropriate amount of fluids/day for the following children.

1. Jenny, who weighs 3 kg
   100 ml/kg/day for each kg up to 10 kg = 100 ml/kg × 3 kg = 300 ml
   Total fluids **300 ml/day**

2. Nahid, who weighs 6 kg
   100 ml/kg/day for each kg up to 10 kg = 100 ml/kg × 6 kg = 600 ml
   Total fluids **600 ml/day**

3. Arkady, who weighs 12 kg
   100 ml/kg/day for each kg up to 10 kg = 100 ml/kg × 10 kg = 1 000 ml plus
   50 ml/kg/day for each additional kg up to 20 kg = 50 ml/kg × 2 kg = 100 ml
   Total fluids **1 100 ml/day**

4. Madeline, who weighs 18 kg
   100 ml/kg/day for each kg up to 10 kg = 100 ml/kg × 10 kg = 1 000 ml plus
   50 ml/kg/day for each additional kg up to 20 kg = 50 ml/kg × 8 kg = 400 ml
   Total fluids **1 400 ml/day**

5. Dagmar, who weighs 24 kg
   100 ml/kg/day for each kg up to 10 kg = 100 ml/kg × 10 kg = 1 000 ml plus
   50 ml/kg/day for each additional kg up to 20 kg = 50 ml/kg × 10 kg = 500 ml plus
   20 ml/kg/day for each additional kg = 20 ml/kg × 4 kg = 80 ml
   Total fluids **1 580 ml/day**

CHAPTER 1

Change these improper fractions to mixed numbers. Reduce the answer to the lowest common denominator.

1. $\dfrac{22}{17} = 1\dfrac{5}{17}$ 2. $\dfrac{15}{12} = 1\dfrac{1}{4}$ 3. $\dfrac{9}{8} = 1\dfrac{1}{8}$ 4. $\dfrac{60}{55} = 1\dfrac{1}{11}$ 5. $\dfrac{66}{30} = 2\dfrac{1}{5}$

Change these mixed numbers to improper fractions. Reduce the answer to the lowest common denominator.

6. $1\dfrac{6}{9} = \dfrac{5}{3}$ 7. $4\dfrac{22}{25} = \dfrac{122}{25}$ 8. $5\dfrac{24}{30} = \dfrac{87}{15}$ 9. $17\dfrac{14}{15} = \dfrac{269}{15}$ 10. $44\dfrac{3}{4} = \dfrac{179}{4}$

For each of the following pairs of fractions, identify which of the two fractions is larger.

11. $\dfrac{3}{4}$ 12. $\dfrac{22}{25}$ 13. $\dfrac{9}{12}$ 14. $\dfrac{12}{15}$ 15. $\dfrac{27}{30}$

Add these fractions. Reduce the answer to the lowest common denominator.

16. $3\dfrac{1}{4} + \dfrac{2}{5} = 3\dfrac{13}{20}$ 17. $\dfrac{6}{9} + \dfrac{9}{12} = 1\dfrac{15}{36}$ 18. $\dfrac{3}{8} + 15\dfrac{11}{12} = 16\dfrac{7}{24}$

19. $\dfrac{22}{30} + \dfrac{5}{6} = 1\dfrac{17}{30}$ 20. $\dfrac{5}{8} + \dfrac{7}{9} = 1\dfrac{29}{72}$

Subtract these fractions. Reduce the answer to the lowest common denominator.

21. $2\dfrac{3}{8} - 1\dfrac{4}{7} = \dfrac{45}{56}$ 22. $5\dfrac{6}{7} - 2\dfrac{5}{9} = 3\dfrac{19}{63}$ 23. $\dfrac{4}{5} - \dfrac{3}{8} = \dfrac{17}{40}$

24. $6\dfrac{11}{12} - 2\dfrac{15}{18} = 4\dfrac{1}{12}$ 25. $4\dfrac{6}{9} - 3\dfrac{4}{6} = 1$

Multiply these fractions. Reduce the answer to the lowest common denominator.

26. $\dfrac{8}{9} \times \dfrac{12}{16} = \dfrac{2}{3}$ 27. $\dfrac{15}{18} \times \dfrac{12}{13} = \dfrac{10}{13}$ 28. $4\dfrac{6}{10} \times \dfrac{17}{19} = 4\dfrac{11}{95}$

29. $\dfrac{18}{20} \times \dfrac{1}{2} = \dfrac{9}{20}$ 30. $5\dfrac{2}{3} \times \dfrac{15}{18} = 4\dfrac{13}{18}$

Divide these fractions. Reduce the answer to the lowest common denominator.

31. $\dfrac{8}{9} \div \dfrac{12}{16} = 1\dfrac{5}{27}$ 32. $\dfrac{15}{18} \div \dfrac{12}{13} = \dfrac{65}{72}$ 33. $4\dfrac{6}{10} \div \dfrac{17}{19} = 5\dfrac{12}{85}$

34. $\dfrac{18}{20} \div \dfrac{1}{2} = 1\dfrac{4}{5}$ 35. $5\dfrac{2}{3} \div \dfrac{15}{18} = 6\dfrac{4}{5}$

Convert these decimals to fractions. Reduce the answer to the lowest common denominator.

36. $1.125 = 1\dfrac{1}{8}$ 37. $5.67 = 5\dfrac{67}{100}$ 38. $15.75 = 15\dfrac{3}{4}$ 39. $0.225 = \dfrac{9}{40}$

40. $0.043 = \dfrac{43}{1\,000}$

Convert these fractions to decimals. State the answer to two decimal places.

41. $\dfrac{1}{2} = 0.5$ 42. $\dfrac{3}{4} = 0.75$ 43. $\dfrac{1}{10} = 0.1$ 44. $\dfrac{13}{15} = 0.87$ 45. $\dfrac{39}{40} = 0.98$

Convert the following decimals to percent. State the answer to one decimal place.

46. $0.25 = $ **25%**   47. $1.75 = $ **175%**   48. $0.03 = $ **3%**   49. $2.04 = $ **204%**

50. $0.009 = $ **0.9%**

Convert these percents to decimals.

51. $3.33\% = $ **0.0333**   52. $0.3\% = $ **0.003**   53. $0.9\% = $ **0.009**

54. $50\% = $ **0.5**   55. $5.25\% = $ **0.0525**

Convert these fractions to percents. State the answer to one decimal place.

56. $\dfrac{1}{3} = $ **33.3%**   57. $\dfrac{1}{8} = $ **12.5%**   58. $\dfrac{1}{6} = $ **16.7%**   59. $\dfrac{2}{3} = $ **66.7%**   60. $\dfrac{3}{5} = $ **60%**

Convert these percents to fractions. Reduce the fraction to its lowest common denominator.

61. $20\% = \dfrac{1}{5}$ 62. $48\% = \dfrac{12}{25}$ 63. $54\% = \dfrac{27}{50}$ 64. $71\% = \dfrac{71}{100}$ 65. $24\% = \dfrac{6}{25}$

CHAPTER 2

You are making a snack mix to take to the hockey banquet. The recipe calls for the following:

125 ml of mixed nuts
200 ml of peanuts
250 ml of garlic-flavoured bite-size bagel chips
750 ml of waffle-shaped corn cereal
500 ml of waffle-shaped wheat cereal
1 000 ml of waffle-shaped rice cereal
90 ml of butter, melted
30 ml of Worcestershire sauce
10 ml of garlic powder
7.5 ml of seasoned salt
2.5 m. of onion powder

Heat the oven to 250°F.
Mix all of the ingredients in a large roast pan.
Bake 1 hour, stirring every 15 minutes.
Spread on paper towels to cool.
Makes 3 000 ml (3 litres) of snack mix.

You decide that you will need 12 000 ml (12 litres) of snack mix for the banquet.

Calculate how much of each of the following ingredients you will need for 12 000 ml of snack mix. Show your calculations using Ratio and Proportion: Means = Extremes and Ratio and Proportion: Cross Multiplication of Fractions.

1. Mixed nuts

Ratio and Proportion: Means = Extremes

The known ratio is 125 ml mixed nuts : 3 000 ml snack mix
The unknown ratio is X ml
mixed nuts : 12 000 ml snack mix
The unknown ratio = the known ratio

$$\downarrow\text{---Means---}\downarrow$$
$$X:12\ 000 \quad = \quad 125:3\ 000\ \text{ml}$$
$$\uparrow\text{---------Extremes----------}\uparrow$$

Means = 1 500 000
Extremes = 3 000 X

Means = Extremes
1 500 000 = 3 000 X

X = 500 ml
You will need **500 ml** of mixed nuts

Ratio and Proportion: Cross Multiplication of Fractions

Known ratio is 125 ml mixed nuts in 3 000 ml snack mix

$$\frac{125}{3\ 000}$$

Unknown ratio is X ml mixed nuts in 12 000 ml snack mix

$$\frac{X}{12\ 000}$$

Unknown ratio = known ratio

$$\frac{X}{12\ 000} = \frac{125}{3\ 000}$$

Cross Multiply

$$\frac{X}{12\ 000} \quad \nwarrow \nearrow \quad \frac{125}{3\ 000}$$

3 000 X = 1 500 000
X = 500
You will need **500 ml** of mixed nuts

2. Peanuts

Ratio and Proportion: Means = Extremes

The known ratio is 200 ml peanuts : 3 000 ml snack mix
The unknown ratio is X ml peanuts : 12 000 ml snack mix
The unknown ratio = the known ratio

$$\downarrow\text{---Means---}\downarrow$$
$$X:12\ 000 \quad = \quad 200:3\ 000\ \text{ml}$$
$$\uparrow\text{---------Extremes----------}\uparrow$$

Means = 2 400 000
Extremes = 3 000 X

Means = Extremes
2 400 000 = 3 000 X

X = 800 ml
You will need **800 ml** of peanuts

Ratio and Proportion: Cross Multiplication of Fractions

Known ratio is 200 ml peanuts in 3 000 ml snack mix

$$\frac{200}{3\ 000}$$

Unknown ratio is X ml peanuts in 12 000 ml snack mix

$$\frac{X}{12\ 000}$$

Unknown ratio = known ratio

$$\frac{X}{12\ 000} = \frac{200}{3\ 000}$$

Cross Multiply

$$\frac{X}{12\ 000} \quad \nwarrow \nearrow \quad \frac{200}{3\ 000}$$

3 000 X = 2 400 000
X = 800
You will need **800 ml** of peanuts

3. Bagel chips

Ratio and Proportion: Means = Extremes

The known ratio is 250 ml
bagel chips : 3 000 ml snack mix
The unknown ratio is X ml
bagel chips : 12 000 ml snack mix
The unknown ratio = the known ratio

$$\downarrow\text{---Means---}\downarrow$$
$$X:12\,000 \;=\; 250:3\,000 \text{ ml}$$
$$\uparrow\text{---------Extremes---------}\uparrow$$

Means = 3 000 000
Extremes = 3 000 X

Means = Extremes
3 000 000 = 3 000 X

X = 1 000 ml
You will need **1 000 ml** of bagel chips

Ratio and Proportion: Cross Multiplication of Fractions

Known ratio is 250 ml bagel chips in 3 000 ml snack mix

$$\frac{250}{3\,000}$$

Unknown ratio is X ml bagel chips in 12 000 ml snack mix

$$\frac{X}{12\,000}$$

Unknown ratio = known ratio

$$\frac{X}{12\,000} = \frac{250}{3\,000}$$

Cross Multiply

$$\frac{X}{12\,000} \;\nwarrow\nearrow\; \frac{250}{3\,000}$$
$$\swarrow\searrow$$

3 000 X = 3 000 000
X = 1 000
You will need **1 000 ml** of bagel chips

4. Corn cereal

Ratio and Proportion: Means = Extremes

The known ratio is 750 ml corn cereal : 3 000 ml snack mix
The unknown ratio is X ml corn cereal : 12 000 ml snack mix
The unknown ratio = the known ratio

$$\downarrow\text{---Means---}\downarrow$$
$$X:12\,000 \;=\; 750:3\,000 \text{ ml}$$
$$\uparrow\text{---------Extremes---------}\uparrow$$

Means = 9 000 000
Extremes = 3 000 X

Means = Extremes
9 000 000 = 3 000 X

X = 3 000 ml
You will need **3 000 ml** of corn cereal

Ratio and Proportion: Cross Multiplication of Fractions

Known ratio is 750 ml corn cereal in 3 000 ml snack mix

$$\frac{750}{3\,000}$$

Unknown ratio is X ml corn cereal in 12 000 ml snack mix

$$\frac{X}{12\,000}$$

Unknown ratio = known ratio

$$\frac{X}{12\,000} = \frac{750}{3\,000}$$

Cross Multiply

$$\frac{X}{12\,000} \;\nwarrow\nearrow\; \frac{750}{3\,000}$$
$$\swarrow\searrow$$

3 000 X = 9 000 000
X = 3 000
You will need **3 000 ml** of corn cereal

5.   Wheat cereal

Ratio and Proportion: Means = Extremes

The known ratio is 500 ml wheat cereal : 3 000 ml snack mix

The unknown ratio is X ml wheat cereal : 12 000 ml snack mix

The unknown ratio = the known ratio

$$\downarrow\text{---Means---}\downarrow$$
$$X:12\,000\quad=\quad500:3\,000\text{ ml}$$
$$\uparrow\text{---------Extremes----------}\uparrow$$

Means = 6 000 000
Extremes = 3 000 X

Means = Extremes
6 000 000 = 3 000 X

X = 2 000 ml
You will need **2 000 ml** of wheat cereal

Ratio and Proportion: Cross Multiplication of Fractions

Known ratio is 500 ml wheat cereal in 3 000 ml snack mix

$$\frac{500}{3\,000}$$

Unknown ratio is X ml wheat cereal in 12 000 ml snack mix

$$\frac{X}{12\,000}$$

Unknown ratio = known ratio

$$\frac{X}{12\,000}=\frac{500}{3\,000}$$

Cross Multiply

$$\frac{X}{12\,000}\quad\nwarrow\quad\nearrow\quad\frac{500}{3\,000}$$
$$\swarrow\quad\searrow$$

3 000 X = 6 000 000
X = 2 000
You will need **2 000 ml** of wheat cereal

6.   Rice cereal

Ratio and Proportion: Means = Extremes

The known ratio is 1 000 ml rice cereal : 3 000 ml snack mix

The unknown ratio is X ml rice cereal : 12 000 ml snack mix

The unknown ratio = the known ratio

$$\downarrow\text{---Means---}\downarrow$$
$$X:12\,000\quad=\quad1\,000:3\,000\text{ ml}$$
$$\uparrow\text{---------Extremes----------}\uparrow$$

Means = 12 000 000
Extremes = 3 000 X

Means = Extremes
12 000 000 = 3 000 X

X = 4 000 ml
You will need **4 000 ml** of rice cereal

Ratio and Proportion: Cross Multiplication of Fractions

Known ratio is 1 000 ml rice cereal in 3 000 ml snack mix

$$\frac{1\,000}{3\,000}$$

Unknown ratio is X ml rice cereal in 12 000 ml snack mix

$$\frac{X}{12\,000}$$

Unknown ratio = known ratio

$$\frac{X}{12\,000}=\frac{1\,000}{3\,000}$$

Cross Multiply

$$\frac{X}{12\,000}\quad\nwarrow\quad\nearrow\quad\frac{1\,000}{3\,000}$$
$$\swarrow\quad\searrow$$

3 000 X = 12 000 000
X = 4 000
You will need **4 000 ml** of rice cereal

7.   Butter

Ratio and Proportion: Means = Extremes

The known ratio is 90 ml butter : 3 000 ml snack mix
The unknown ratio is X ml butter : 12 000 ml snack mix
The unknown ratio = the known ratio

$$\downarrow\text{---Means---}\downarrow$$
$$X:12\,000 \quad = \quad 90:3\,000\text{ ml}$$
$$\uparrow\text{---------Extremes---------}\uparrow$$

Means = 1 080 000
Extremes = 3 000 X

Means = Extremes
1 080 000 = 3 000 X

X = 360 ml
You will need **360 ml** of butter

Ratio and Proportion: Cross Multiplication of Fractions

Known ratio is 90 ml butter in 3 000 ml snack mix

$$\frac{90}{3\,000}$$

Unknown ratio is X ml butter in 12 000 ml snack mix

$$\frac{X}{12\,000}$$

Unknown ratio = known ratio

$$\frac{X}{12\,000} = \frac{90}{3\,000}$$

Cross Multiply

$$\frac{X}{12\,000} \quad \nwarrow \nearrow \quad \frac{90}{3\,000}$$
$$\swarrow \searrow$$

3 000 X = 1 080 000
X = 360
You will need **360 ml** of butter

8.   Worcestershire sauce

Ratio and Proportion: Means = Extremes

The known ratio is
30 ml Worcestershire sauce: 3 000 ml snack mix
The unknown ratio is
X ml Worcestershire sauce : 12 000 ml snack mix
The unknown ratio = the known ratio

$$\downarrow\text{---Means---}\downarrow$$
$$X:12\,000 \quad = \quad 30:3\,000\text{ ml}$$
$$\uparrow\text{---------Extremes---------}\uparrow$$

Means = 360 000
Extremes = 3 000 X

Means = Extremes
360 000 = 3 000 X

X = 120 ml
You will need **120 ml** of Worcestershire sauce

Ratio and Proportion: Cross Multiplication of Fractions

Known ratio is 30 ml Worcestershire sauce in 3 000 ml snack mix

$$\frac{30}{3\,000}$$

Unknown ratio is X ml Worcestershire sauce in 12 000 ml snack mix

$$\frac{X}{12\,000}$$

Unknown ratio = known ratio

$$\frac{X}{12\,000} = \frac{30}{3\,000}$$

Cross Multiply

$$\frac{X}{12\,000} \quad \nwarrow \nearrow \quad \frac{30}{3\,000}$$
$$\swarrow \searrow$$

3 000 X = 360 000
X = 120
You will need **120 ml** of Worcestershire sauce

9. Garlic powder

Ratio and Proportion: Means = Extremes

The known ratio is 10 ml garlic powder : 3 000 ml snack mix
The unknown ratio is X ml garlic powder : 12 000 ml snack mix
The unknown ratio = the known ratio

$$\downarrow\text{---Means---}\downarrow$$
$$X:12\ 000\quad =\quad 10:3\ 000\ ml$$
$$\uparrow\text{--------Extremes--------}\uparrow$$

Means = 120 000
Extremes = 3 000 X

Means = Extremes
120 000 = 3 000 X

X = 40 ml
You will need **40 ml** of garlic powder

Ratio and Proportion: Cross Multiplication of Fractions

Known ratio is 10 ml garlic powder in 3 000 ml snack mix

$$\frac{10}{3\ 000}$$

Unknown ratio is X ml garlic powder in 12 000 ml snack mix

$$\frac{X}{12\ 000}$$

Unknown ratio = known ratio

$$\frac{X}{12\ 000} = \frac{10}{3\ 000}$$

Cross Multiply

$$\frac{X}{12\ 000} \quad\nwarrow\ \nearrow\quad \frac{10}{3\ 000}$$

3 000 X = 120 000
X = 40
You will need **40 ml** of garlic powder

10. Seasoned salt

Ratio and Proportion: Means = Extremes

The known ratio is 7.5 ml seasoned salt : 3 000 ml snack mix
The unknown ratio is X ml seasoned salt : 12 000 ml snack mix
The unknown ratio = the known ratio

$$\downarrow\text{---Means---}\downarrow$$
$$X:12\ 000\quad =\quad 7.5:3\ 000\ ml$$
$$\uparrow\text{--------Extremes--------}\uparrow$$

Means = 90 000
Extremes = 3 000 X

Means = Extremes
90 000 = 3 000 X

X = 30 ml
You will need **30 ml** of seasoned salt

Ratio and Proportion: Cross Multiplication of Fractions

Known ratio is 7.5 ml of seasoned salt in 3 000 ml snack mix

$$\frac{7.5}{3\ 000}$$

Unknown ratio is X ml seasoned salt in 12 000 ml snack mix

$$\frac{X}{12\ 000}$$

Unknown ratio = known ratio

$$\frac{X}{12\ 000} = \frac{7.5}{3\ 000}$$

Cross Multiply

$$\frac{X}{12\ 000} \quad\nwarrow\ \nearrow\quad \frac{7.5}{3\ 000}$$

3 000 X = 90 000
X = 30
You will need **30 ml** of seasoned salt

11. Onion powder

Ratio and Proportion: Means = Extremes	**Ratio and Proportion: Cross Multiplication of Fractions**
The known ratio is 2.5 ml onion powder : 3 000 ml snack mix The unknown ratio is X ml onion powder : 12 000 ml snack mix The unknown ratio = the known ratio	Known ratio is 2.5 ml onion powder in 3 000 ml snack mix

Ratio and Proportion: Means = Extremes

The known ratio is 2.5 ml onion powder : 3 000 ml snack mix
The unknown ratio is X ml onion powder : 12 000 ml snack mix
The unknown ratio = the known ratio

$$\downarrow\text{---Means---}\downarrow$$
$$X:12\,000 \quad = \quad 2.5:3\,000 \text{ ml}$$
$$\uparrow\text{---------Extremes---------}\uparrow$$

Means = 30 000
Extremes = 3 000 X

Means = Extremes
30 000 = 3 000 X

X = 10 ml
You will need **10 ml** of onion powder

Ratio and Proportion: Cross Multiplication of Fractions

Known ratio is 2.5 ml onion powder in 3 000 ml snack mix

$$\frac{2.5}{3\,000}$$

Unknown ratio is X ml onion powder in 12 000 ml snack mix

$$\frac{X}{12\,000}$$

Unknown ratio = known ratio

$$\frac{X}{12\,000} = \frac{2.5}{3\,000}$$

Cross Multiply

$$\frac{X}{12\,000} \quad \nwarrow \nearrow \quad \frac{2.5}{3\,000}$$
$$\swarrow \searrow$$

3 000 X = 30 000
X = 10
You will need **10 ml** of onion powder

CHAPTER 3

Write out each of the following in full:

1. Tylenol (acetaminophen) elix 80 mg per NG q4h prn.

   Tylenol (acetaminophen) elixir 80 milligrams, by nasogastric tube, every four hours, as necessary.

2. Cardizem CD (diltiazem) 160 mg po qam.

   Cardizem controlled delivery (diltiazem) 160 milligrams, by mouth, every morning.

3. Ativan 0.5 mg sl qhs.

   Ativan 0.5 milligrams, sublingually, every evening.

4. Voltaren Opthalmic 1% sol (diclofenac) gtts ĩ OS qid × 1 week then bid × 1 week.

   Voltaren Opthalmic 1% solution (diclofenac) one drop, in the left eye, four times per day, for one week, then two times daily, for one week.

5. Alti-Beclomethasone (beclomethasone) MDI 2 puffs q8h.

   Alti-Beclomethasone (beclomethasone) by metered dose inhaler, 2 puffs, every 8 hours.

6. Dilaudid (hydromorphone) 4 mg IM q3h prn.

   Dilaudid (hydromorphone) 4 milligrams, intramuscularly, every 3 hours, as necessary.

Write out each of the following using the abbreviations in Chapters 3.

7. Canesten (nystatin) suppository 1 gram into the vagina at bedtime.

   Canesten (nystatin) supp 1 g PV qhs.

8. Nu-Ranit (ranitidine) 150 milligrams by mouth twice daily.

   Nu-Ranit (ranitidine) 150 mg po bid.

9. Ceruminex (triethanolamine polypeptide oleate-condensate) 1 millilitre in each ear at bedtime.

   Ceruminex (triethanolamine polypeptide oleate-condensate) 1 ml AU qhs.

10. Apo-Cefaclor (cefaclor) suspension 250 milligrams by mouth three times each day.

    Apo-Cefaclor (cefaclor) susp 250 mg po tid.

11. Lasix (furosemide) 40 milligrams intravenously, immediately.

    Lasix (furosemide) 40 mg IV stat.

12. Heparin (heparin) 5 000 international units subcutaneously every morning and evening.

    Heparin (heparin) 5 000 iu sc qam and qhs.

CHAPTER 4

Identify which of the following are correct according to the rules of SI usage. For those that are not, write the correct form in the following space.

1. Centigram

   centigram

2. 1,000,000

   1 000 000

3. 10mg

   10 mg

4. 15 kg

   correct

5. 25 l

   25 L

Change the following amounts from grams (g) to milligrams (mg).

6. 0.05 g

   50 mg

7. 2.3 g

   2 300 mg

8. 0.4 g

   400 mg

9. 1.2 g

   1 200 mg

10. 0.006 g

    6 mg

Change the following amounts from milligrams (mg) to grams (g).

11. 25 mg

    0.025 g

12. 200 mg

    0.2 g

13. 1 mg

    0.001 g

14. 1 200 mg

    1.2 g

15. 500 mg

    0.5 g

Change the following amounts from micrograms (mcg or μg) to milligrams (mg)

16. 1 mcg

    0.001 mg

17. 250 μg

    0.25 mg

18. 100 μg

    0.1 mg

19. 40 mcg

    0.04 mg

20. 600 μg

    0.6 mg

Change the following amounts from milligrams (mg) to micrograms (mcg or μg)

21. 1 mg

    1 000 μg

22. 0.005 mg

    5 mcg

23. 0.0007 mg

    0.7 mcg

24. 20 mg

    20 000 μg

25. 0.025 mg

_____25 mcg_____

MULTIPLE CHOICE QUESTIONS

26. A mole is a measurement of which of the following?

   C. *The amount of a substance that contains the same number of particles as there are atoms in 12 g of carbon-12.*

27. A grain is a measurement of which of the following?

   D. *The unit of weight in the apothecary system.*

28. A unit is a measurement of which of the following?

   B. *An internationally agreed-upon amount that has a specific biological effect.*

29. An equivalent is a measurement of which of the following?

   A. *The amount of a substance that will combine with 1 g of hydrogen.*

30. It is after noon and you check your watch to discover the time. Identify the 24-hour clock time for each of the watch faces below.

30a.

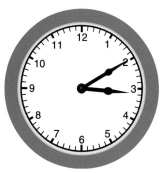

_____1510 hrs_____

30b.

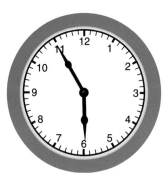

_____1755 hrs_____

30c.

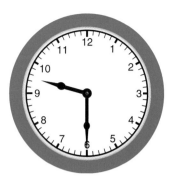

_____2130 hrs_____

30d.

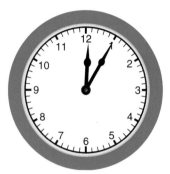

_____1205 hrs_____

30e.

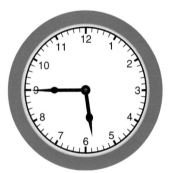

_____1745 hrs_____

CHAPTER 5

1. Which of the following doctor's orders must be signed by the physician?

    D. All doctor's orders

2. Identify which of the following represent a functional classification and which of the following represent a chemical classification:

    A. β blockers—chemical

    B. Antihypertensives—functional

C. Antianginals—functional

D. ACE inhibitors—chemical

3. Which of the following liquid medications contain alcohol?

   A. Elixir   and   D. Fluid extract

4. Enteric-coated tablets are designed to dissolve in which of the following parts of the GI tract?

   C. Duodenum

5. Your patient has an order for *morphine 5 mg any route q2h prn*. She states that she is having severe pain. You feel that it is important that she get relief from her pain as quickly as possible. Which of the following routes will you choose?

   A. Intravenous

6. Your patient has an order for *Maxeran (metoclopramide) 10 mg po qid AC and HS*. When will you give this drug?

   You will determine the times that meals are served and give the Maxeran $\frac{1}{2}$ hour before each meal. You will give the HS dose at bedtime, usually 2100 or 2200 hours.

7. Identify the omissions in the doctor's orders that are shown in Figure 5.8.

   No route for celecoxib

   No time/frequency for Ventolin

   No dose for Zinacef

   No time/frequency for laxative. Laxative orders are also usually prn.

   No doctor's signature

CHAPTER 6

1. What is the generic name of this drug?

   pantoprazole sodium

2. What is the adult dosage range?

   20–40 mg

3. What is the strength of the tablets?

   40 mg

4. What is the expiry date?

   January 2006

5. Who should not take this drug?

   Pregnant women, women who are nursing, children.

6. Who manufactured this drug?

   Solvay Pharma Inc., Markham, Ontario, L3R 0C9

7. What preparation are these tablets?

   Enteric coated tablets

8. Where should these tablets be stored?

   Controlled room temperature (15–30°C)

9. What is the lot number of this package?

   135976

10. What class of drug is this?

    H⁺, K⁺ -ATPase Inhibitor

CHAPTER 7

1. Identify the components of a Medication Administration Record.

   the name of the patient

   any medication allergies

   drug name

   dose

   route

   frequency

   any special instruction

2. Which system provides a 24-hour supply of medication?

   Unit dose

3. Which system usually provides a week's supply of medication?

   Individual bottles

4. Which system poses the greatest risk of error?

   Stock supply

5. Which system may be used to supplement other systems?

   Stock supply

CHAPTER 8

ORAL SOLIDS

In the space below the question, write the number of tablets or capsules you will give in order to administer the medication as written.

1. Doctor's order *Prevacid 30 mg.* Stock **Prevacid 15 mg tablets.**

   2 tab

2. Doctor's order *Levodopa 150 mg.* Stock **Levodopa 100 mg tablets.**

   1¹/₂ tab

3. Doctor's order *Librium 30 mg.* Stock **Librium 10 mg capsules.**

   3 cap

4. Doctor's order *dimenhydrinate 25 mg*. Stock **dimenhydrenate 50 mg tablets**.

   _____1/2 tab_____

5. Doctor's order *Diabenase 125 mg*. Stock **Diabenase 250 mg tablets**.

   _____1/2 tab_____

6. Doctor's order *Ceftin 1 gm*. Stock **Ceftin 500 mg capsules**.

   _____2 cap_____

7. Doctor's order *Digoxin 0.125 mg*. Stock **Digoxin 0.25 mg tablets**.

   _____1/2 tab_____

8. Doctor's order *Digoxin 0.5 mg*. Stock **Digoxin 0.25 mg tablets**.

   _____2 tab_____

9. Doctor's order *Digoxin 0.0625 mg*. Stock **Digoxin 0.125 mg tablets**.

   _____1/2 tab_____

10. Doctor's order *Penicillin G 1 million units*. Stock **Penicillin G 500 000 unit tablets**.

    _____2 tab_____

ORAL LIQUIDS

In the space below the question, write the number of ml you will give to comply with the order.

11. Doctor's order *Colace 100 mg*. Stock **Colace syrup 20 mg/5 ml**.

    _____25 ml_____

12. Doctor's order *Zithromax 600 mg*. Stock **Zithromax suspension 900 mg/22.5 ml**.

    _____15 ml_____

13. Doctor's order *Erythrocin 750 mg*. Stock **Erythrocin suspension 250 mg/5 ml**.

    _____15 ml_____

14. Doctor's order *Apo-Cloxi 200 mg*. Stock **Apo-Cloxi suspension 125 mg/5 ml**.

    _____8 ml_____

15. Doctor's order *Amoxil 600 mg*. Stock **Amoxil Suspension 250 mg/5 ml**.

    _____12 ml_____

16. Doctor's order *Gravol 25 mg*. Stock **Gravol liquid 15 mg/5 ml**.

    _____8.3 ml_____

17. Doctor's order *Benadryl 12.5 mg*. Stock **Benadryl Elixir 6.25 mg/5 ml**.

    _____10 ml_____

18. Doctor's order *dicyclomine 15 mg*. Stock **dicyclomine syrup 10 mg/5 ml**.

    _____7.5 ml_____

19. Doctor's order *Kaon 40 mEq*. Stock **Kaon liquid 20 mEq/15 ml**.

    _____30 ml_____

20. Doctor's order *Periactin 20 mg*. Stock **Periactin Syrup 2 mg/5 ml**.

    _____50 ml_____

CHAPTER 9

In the space below the questions, write the number of ml you will give.

1. Doctor's order *Isoptin (verapamil) 7.5 mg slow IV push stat.* Stock **Verapamil 2.5 mg/2 ml.**

    _____6 ml_____

2. Doctor's order *Dilantin (phenytoin) 100 mg IM Q4H × 24 hours.* Stock **phenytoin injection 50 mg/ml.**

    _____2 ml_____

3. Doctor's order *thiamine 100 mg IM QAM.* Stock **thiamine 1 000 mg/10 ml.**

    _____1 ml_____

4. Doctor's order *Toradol (keterolac) 25 mg IM Q4H PRN.* Stock **Toradol 30 mg/ml.**

    _____0.8 ml_____

5. Doctor's order *gentamycin 60 mg IV Q8H.* Stock **gentamycin 40 mg/ml.**

    _____1.5 ml_____

6. Doctor's order *morphine 12 mg SC Q3H PRN.* Stock **morphine 15 mg/ml.**

    _____0.8 ml_____

7. Doctor's order *Stemetil (prochlorperazine) 2.5 mg IM Q4H PRN.* Stock **Stemetil 10 mg/2ml.**

    _____0.5 ml_____

8. Doctor's order *Vitamin B$_{12}$ 2 mg IM each month.* Stock **Vitamin B$_{12}$ 1 000 mcg/ml.**

    _____2 ml_____

9. Doctor's order *Demerol (meperidine) 125 mg IM Q3H PRN.* Stock **Demerol 75 mg/ml.**

    _____1.7 ml_____

10. Doctor's order *Dilaudid (hydromorphone) 1 mg Q2H PRN.* Stock **hydromorphone 2 mg/ml.**

    _____0.5 ml_____

In the space below the questions, write the number of ml you will give.

11. Doctor's order *Maxipime (cefepime) 0.5 g IM Q12H × 7 days.* Stock **Maxipime 1 g vial.** Add 2.4 ml sterile water for injection. Approximate concentration 280 mg/ml.

    _____1.8 ml_____

12. Doctor's order *Zinacef (cefuroxime) 1 g IV Q8H.* Stock **Zinacef 750 mg vials.** Add 8 ml sterile water for injection. Approximate concentration 90 mg/ml.

    _____11 ml_____

13. Doctor's order *Fortaz (ceftazidime)1.5 g IV Q12H* . Stock **Fortaz 1 g vials.** Add 10 ml sterile water for injection. Approximate concentration 100 mg/ml.

    _____*15 ml*_____

14. Doctor's order *Ancef (cefazolin) 1 g IV Q8H*. Stock **Ancef 500 mg vials.** Add 2. ml sodium chloride for injection. Approximate concentration 225 mg/ml.

    _____*4.4 ml*_____

15. Doctor's order *Zovirax (acyclovir) 600 mg IV Q8H × 7 days*. Stock **Zovirax 1 g vial.** Add 20 ml sterile water for injection. Approximate concentration 50 mg/ml.

    _____*12 ml*_____

CHAPTER 12

Calculate the drip rate for the following gravity IVs.

1. Doctor's order reads *IV NS 3 000 ml per day.* Drip factor is 10.

   _____*21 gtts/min*_____

2. Doctor's order reads *IV 1 000 ml over the next 6 hours.* Drip factor is 15.

   _____*42 gtts/min*_____

3. Doctor's order reads *IV D5W 1 000 ml per shift.* The shift is 8 hours. Drip factor is 15.

   _____*31 gtts/min*_____

4. Doctor's order reads *IV Ringer's Lactate 60 ml per hour.* Drip factor is 12.

   _____*12 gtts/min*_____

5. Doctor's order reads *IV 2/3 + 1/3 1 500 ml/shift.* The shift is 12 hours. Drip factor is 12.

   _____*25 gtts/min*_____

Calculate the drip rate for the following gravity IVs with microdrip tubing.

6. Doctor's order reads *IV 2/3 + 1/3 500 ml Q8H.*

   _____*62.5 gtts/min*_____

7. Doctor's order reads *IV D5W 2 000 ml Q24H.*

   _____*83 gtts/min*_____

8. Doctor's order reads *IV D5W 600 ml Q8H*

   _____*75 gtts/min*_____

9. Doctor's order reads *IV NS 40 ml/hr.*

   _____*40 gtts/min*_____

10. Doctor's order reads *IV Ringer's Lactate 50 ml/hr.*

    _____*50 gtts/min*_____

Calculate the flow rate for the following IV orders which are to be administered using an IV pump.

11. Doctor's order reads *IV NS 1 000 ml Q6H.*

    _____167 ml/hr_____

12. Doctor's order reads *IV Ringer's Lactate 1 000 ml Q8H.*

    _____125 ml/hr_____

13. Doctor's order reads *IV Normosol M 1 000 ml Q12H.*

    _____83 ml/hr_____

14. Doctor's order reads *IV D5W 1 500 ml Q8H.*

    _____188 ml/hr_____

15. Doctor's order reads *IV NS 500 ml Q12H.*

    _____42 ml/hr_____

CHAPTER 13

Calculate the drip rate for the following IV medications. The medications are added to a minibag that is used with a gravity IV.

1. Doctor's order reads *metronidazole 100 mg IV Q8H.* The metronidazole comes premixed in a 100 ml minibag and is to be administered over 45 minutes. The drip factor is 12.

    _____27 gtts/min_____

2. Doctor's order reads *Lasix 40 mg IV stat.* The label on the vial reads Lasix 40 mg/4ml. You decide to mix the Lasix in a 50 ml bag and administer it over 20 minutes. The drip factor is 15.

    _____40 gtts/min_____

3. Doctor's order reads *Rocephin 1 g IV Q12H.* When reconstituted, there is 1 g of Rocephin in 10 ml of solution. You decide to dilute it in 100 ml of normal saline and administer it over 1 hour. The drip factor is 15.

    _____28 gtts/min_____

4. Doctor's order reads *Zinacef 1.5 g IV Q8H.* When reconstituted, there is 1.5 g of Zinacef in 16 ml of solution. You decide to dilute it in 50 ml of normal saline and administer it over 30 minutes. The drip factor is 10.

    _____22 gtts/min_____

5. Doctor's order reads is *ranitidine 50 mg IV QHS.* The ranitidine is in a vial labelled 25 mg/ml. You decide to dilute it in 50 ml of normal saline and administer it over 25 minutes. The drip factor is 15.

    _____31 gtts/min_____

Calculate the flow rate for the following IV medications. The medications are added to a minibag and administered using an IV pump.

6. Doctor's order reads *Cipro (ciprofloxacin) 400 mg IV Q12H*. Cipro must be diluted in 250 mg of normal saline. You decide to administer it over 90 minutes.

   ___167 ml/hr___

7. Doctor's order reads *Pantoloc (patoprazole) 40 mg IV QHS*. When reconstituted, there are 40 mg of Pantoloc in 10 ml of solution. It should be further diluted in 100 ml of normal saline and administered over 1 hour.

   ___110 ml/hr___

8. Doctor's order reads *Solu-Medrol (methylprednisolone) 500 mg IV Q8H*. When reconstituted, there are 500 mg of Solu-Medrol in 8 ml of solution. You decide to dilute it in 50 ml of normal saline and administer it over 30 minutes.

   ___116 ml/hr___

9. Doctor's order reads *vancomycin 1 g IV Q8H*. When reconstituted there is 1 g of vancomycin in 20 ml of solution. This must be further diluted in 250 ml of normal saline and administered over 60 minutes.

   ___270 ml/hr___

10. Doctor's order reads *Ancef (cefazolin) 1 g IV Q8H*. When reconstituted there is 1 g of Ancef in 3 ml of solution. You decide to dilute it in 50 ml of normal saline and administer it over 20 minutes.

    ___159 ml/hr___

Calculate the drip rate for the following IV medications. The medications are added to a soluset.

11. Doctor's order reads *gentamycin 40 mg IV Q8H*. Gentamycin is supplied in a concentration of 40 mg/ml. You decide to further dilute it to 125 ml of fluid and to administer it over 90 minutes.

    ___83 gtts/min___

12. Doctor's order reads *clindamycin 600 mg IV Q6H*. Clindamycin is supplied in 4 ml vials which have a strength of 150 mg/ml. The package states that you should further dilute it to 50 ml of compatible IV solution and administer it over 20 minutes.

    ___150 gtts/min___

13. Doctor's order reads *Rocephin (ceftriaxone) 1 g IV Q12H*. When reconstituted, there is 1 g of Rocephin in 10 ml of solution. You decide to further dilute it to 75 ml of fluid and administer it over 45 minutes.

    ___100 gtts/min___

14. Doctor's order reads *Cefizox (ceftizoxime) 2 g IV Q12H*. When reconstituted, there is 2 g of Cefizox in 20 ml of solution. You decide to further dilute it to 70 ml of fluid and administer it over 75 minutes.

    ___56 gtts/min___

15. Doctor's order reads *dimenhydrinate 50 mg IV Q4H PRN for nausea.* Dimenhydrinate is supplied in a concentration of 50 mg/ml. You decide to further dilute it to 30 ml of fluid and to administer it over 15 minutes.

     120 gtts/min

Calculate the flow rate for the following medications administered using an IV pump.

16. Doctor's order reads *magnesium sulphate IV 1 g/hour × 24 hours.* Your drug guide tells you to mix 25 g of magnesium sulphate in 250 ml of D5W.

     10 ml/hr

17. Doctor's order reads *Pantoloc (pantoprazole) IV 8 mg/hour.* Pharmacy sends you a 100 ml bag that has a concentration of 0.4 mg/ml.

     20 ml/hr

18. Doctor's order reads *amiodarone IV 1 mg/min.* Hospital policy states that you will mix 450 mg of amiodarone in 250 ml of D5W.

     33 ml/hr

19. Doctor's order reads *amiodarone IV 15 mg/min for 10 min for breakthrough arrhythmia.* Hospital policy states that you will mix 450 mg of amiodarone in 250 ml of D5W.

     500 ml/hr

20. Doctor's order reads *theophylline IV 0.5 mg/kg/hr.* Theophylline comes in a pre-mixed bag of 500 mg/500 ml of D5W. The patient's weight is 68 kg.

     34 ml/hr

CHAPTER 14

CASE STUDY

Mrs. Evelyn Maracle is a 57-year-old woman who has recently been diagnosed with NIDDM, or Type 2 diabetes mellitus. She has been reluctant to accept this diagnosis and admits to being noncompliant with her diet. She has been admitted to your hospital floor with a blood sugar of 39 mmol/L. Her doctor's orders are as follows.

Insulin IV 12 u/hr until 0700 hrs tomorrow.
NPH insulin 22 u sc ½ hr ac breakfast
NPH insulin 16 u sc ½ ac supper
Glucometer TID ½ hour ac meals and HS

> Glucometer   < 9.9 no insulin
> 10.0–12.9 give 6 units regular insulin
> 13.0–15.9 give 9 units regular insulin
> 16.0–18.9 give 11 units regular insulin
> 19.0–21.9 give 13 units regular insulin
> > 22 call for further orders

The IV insulin is in a premixed bag with a strength of 125 u of insulin in 250 ml of NS. Hospital policy in your institution states that IV insulin is always administered using a pump.

1. At what rate will you run the IV?

   24 ml/hr

2. Mrs. Maracle's glucometer readings have been recorded on the diabetic record below. Using those readings, document all of the insulin that should be administered over the next 2 days.

Init	Signature
AZ	Alan Zaicsky RPN
CR	Carla Ramirez RN

AGH
Anywhere General Hospital
DIABETIC
RECORD

5723753

Maracle, Evelyn
546 Front St.
Apt. 448
Anywhere,
Ontario

Allergies   *NKA*

Diagnosis *NIDDM*
Arterial Insufficiency

Date Time	Glucometer	Insulin by Reaction	Scheduled Insulin	Init
06/10/04 0730	14.7	Regular Insulin 9 u sc	NPH Insulin 22 u sc	AZ
1130	10.2	Regular Insulin 6 u sc		AZ
1630	16.3	Regular Insulin 11 u sc	NPH Insulin 16 u sc	CR
2200	7.1			
07/10/04 0730	19.4	Regular Insulin 13 u sc	NPH Insulin 22 u sc	AZ
1130	12.3	Regular Insulin 6 u sc		AZ
1630	14.1	Regular Insulin 9 u sc	NPH Insulin 16 u sc	CR
2200	8.8			

3. On the syringes below, identify the time and amounts of each *mixed* insulin that should be given as a result of the above doctor's orders and glucometer readings.

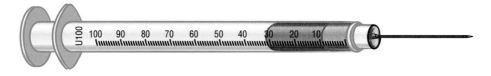

Regular insulin 9 u plus NPH insulin 22 u

Total insulin 31 u

Time 0730 hrs 06/10/04

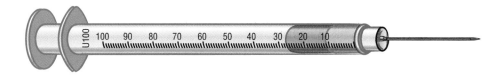

Regular insulin 11 u plus NPH insulin 16 u

Total insulin 27 u

Time 1630 hrs 06/10/04

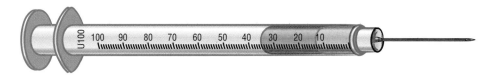

Regular insulin 13 u plus NPH insulin 22 u

Total insulin 35 u

Time 0730 hrs 07/10/04

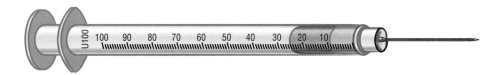

Regular insulin 9 u plus NPH insulin 16 u

Total insulin 25 u

Time 1630 hrs 07/10/04

CHAPTER 15

CASE STUDY

Elizabeth Komarovsky is a 38-year-old woman who has been admitted with a pulmonary embolus. She weighs 54 kg. Her heparin orders are as follows:

Heparin IV at 90 u/kg/hr until APPT is 2 times control, then
Heparin IV at 20 u/kg/hr to maintain target APPT

Heparin is supplied premixed with 25 000 u of heparin in 250 ml of normal saline.

1. At what rate will you run the IV on admission?

    _____49 ml/hr_____

2. At what rate will you run the IV when the target APPT is reached?

    _____11 ml/hr_____

Mrs. Komarovsky's physician is monitoring her APPT twice daily. Her APPT starts to rise so he changes the order to *Heparin IV at 17 u/kg/hr.*

3. At what rate will you run the IV?

    9 ml/hr

Three days later, the physician decides to change her heparin to subcutaneous injection. The order now reads *Heparin 9 000 u sc BID*. The heparin is in an ampoule labelled **Heparin 10 000 u/ml**.

4. How much heparin will you draw up?

    0.9 ml

After a week of heparin therapy, the physician decides to change to Coumadin. The order reads *Coumadin 3 mgm* today. You look in the medication cupboard and find that there are bottles of **Coumadin 1 mg tablets, Coumadin 2 mg tablets**, and **Coumadin 5 mg tablets** available.

5. What combination of tablets will you pour for Mrs. Komarovsky?

    One 1 mg tablet and one 2 mg tablet

CHAPTER 16

DRUG AND SAFE DOSE CALCULATIONS

1. Jenna weighs 13 kg. The doctor's order reads *Apo-Cloxi (cloxicillin) 20 mg/kg po q6h*. Maximum safe dose is 4 g/day. The label on the bottle reads **Apo-Cloxi Suspension 125 mg/5ml**. How many mg of Apo-Cloxi will you give? How much Apo-Cloxi will you pour? How will you measure it? Is this within the safe dosage range?

    260 mg Apo-Cloxi per dose

    10.4 ml

    The dose is within the safe dosage range.

2. Andrew weighs 22 kg. The doctor's order reads *rifampin 300 mg po daily*. The label on the bottle reads **rifampin 150 mg capsules.** The safe dosage range is 10–20 mg/kg/day. How many capsules will you administer? Is this dose within the safe range?

    2 capsules

    The dose is within the safe dosage range.

3. Marcel weighs 38 kg and is 140 cm tall. The doctor's order reads *Amicar (aminocaproic acid) 5 g IV, followed by 1 g q1h until bleeding is controlled*. The label on the vial reads **Amicar 250 mg/ml.** The maximum safe dose is 18 g/m²/24 hours. How much Amicar will you draw up for the first dose? How much will you draw up for each subsequent dose? If the bleeding continues for 24 hours, will the maximum safe dosage range be exceeded?

    20 ml Amicar for the first dose

    4 ml of Amicar for the subsequent doses

Marcel's BSA is 1.2 m². The maximum safe dose for him is 21.6 gm. In 24 hours he would receive 28 gm of Amicar. This is outside the usual safe dosage range.

4. Alice weighs 15 kg. The doctor's order reads *Septra (trimethoprim/sulfamethoxa-zole) 5 ml IV q6h.* The safe dosage range for Septra is 0.31–0.63 ml/kg. Is this dose within the safe range?

   The dose is within the safe range.

5. Thea weighs 9 kg. The doctor's order reads *penicillin G 125 000 u IV q4h.* The label on the vial reads **penicillin G 1 000 000 u.** It is to be reconstituted with 3 ml of sterile water. How much penicillin will you draw up? The safe dosage range for penicillin G is 25 000–300 000 u/kg in 24 hours. Is this dose within the safe range?

   0.38 ml of penicillin

   The dose is within the safe range.

FLUID INTAKE CALCULATIONS

Calculate the appropriate fluid intake for the following children.

1. Helena, who weighs 4.7 kg

   470 ml

2. Anneka, who weighs 7.7 kg

   770 ml

3. Robby, who weighs 11.4 kg

   1 070 ml

4. Jamie, who weighs 16.2 kg

   1 310 ml

5. Kayla, who weighs 18.4 kg

   1 420 ml

6. Shawna, who weighs 22.5 kg

   1 550 ml

7. Lili, who weighs 24 kg

   1 580 ml

8. Pierre, who weighs 25.8 kg

   1 616 ml

9. Gurmant, who weighs 28 kg

   1 660 ml

10. Elizabeth, who weighs 35 kg

    1 800 ml

CASE STUDY

Andrew is a 5-year-old boy who is being treated for exacerbation of acute lymphocytic leukemia. He is 110 cm tall and weighs 16 kg. His doctor's orders are as follows:

AGH Anywhere General Hospital	0239705 Zaleski, Andrew 44 Coleman St. Apt 16 Anywhere, Ontario

Doctor's Orders

Date	Orders
Feb 2/05	Days 1–7 inclusive
	Cytostar 100 mg/m² IV od
	Days 1–3 inclusive
	Adriamycin 30 mg/m² IV od
	Days 1–5 inclusive
	Solu–cortef 40 mg/m² IV bid
	Days 1 and 5
	vincristine 1.5 mg/m² od
	A.K. Gryffe MD

The labels on the medication containers read as follows:

Cytostar (cytarabine) 100 mg vial. Dilute with 5 ml of NS for a concentration of 20 mg/ml

Adriamycin (doxyrubacin) 50 mg/25 ml

Solu-cortef (hydrocortisone) Act-O-Vial. When mixed, each vial contains 100 mg/2 ml

Vincristine 1 mg/ml in each 2-ml vial

Identify which drugs you will give on each day of this 7-day course of chemotherapy. Identify the dose of the drug, and the amount of solution you will draw up.

Andrew must be well-hydrated during this course of chemotherapy. How much fluid should he have each day?

Day 1
Cytostar (cytarabine) **70 mg** IV od
Draw up **3.5 ml**

Adriamycin (doxyrubacin) **21 mg** IV od
Draw up **10.5 ml**

Solu-cortef (hydrocortisone) **28 mg** IV bid
Draw up **0.56 ml**

Vincristine **1.1 mg** IV od
Draw up **1.1 ml**

Day 2
Cytostar (cytarabine) **70 mg** IV od
Draw up **3.5 ml**

Adriamycin (doxyrubacin) **21 mg** IV od
Draw up **10.5 ml**

Solu-cortef (hydrocortisone) **28 mg** IV bid
Draw up **0.56 ml**

Day 3
Cytostar (cytarabine) **70 mg** IV od
Draw up **3.5 ml**

Adriamycin (doxyrubacin) **21 mg** IV od
Draw up **10.5 ml**

Solu-cortef (hydrocortisone) **28 mg** IV bid
Draw up **0.56 ml**

Day 4
Cytostar (cytarabine) **70 mg** IV od
Draw up **3.5 ml**

Solu-cortef (hydrocortisone) **28 mg** IV bid
Draw up **0.56 ml**

Day 5
Cytostar (cytarabine) **70 mg** IV od
Draw up **3.5 ml**

Solu-cortef (hydrocortisone) **28 mg** IV bid
Draw up **0.56 ml**

Vincristine **1.1 mg** IV od
Draw up **1.1 ml**

Day 6
Cytostar (cytarabine) **70 mg** IV od
Draw up **3.5 ml**

Day 7
Cytostar (cytarabine) **70 mg IV od**
Draw up **3.5 ml**

Andrew's fluid intake should be at least 1 300 ml/day.

CHAPTER 17

Match the potential complication associated with blood transfusion with the measures usually taken to prevent them.

1. Haemolytic reaction—C
2. Febrile reaction—E
3. Bacterial contamination—B
4. Allergic reaction—A
5. Fluid volume excess—D
6. What is the only IV solution that can be administered with blood?

    Normal saline

7. Which blood component has a lifespan of only 5 days?

    Platelets

8. Which blood component can cause a significant shift of fluid from the abdominal cavity into the vascular system?

    Albumin

9. Identify the components of the nursing assessment that should be carried out on any patient who is receiving a transfusion of blood or blood products.

    - Vital signs
      - temperature
      - pulse
      - respirations
      - blood pressure
    - Chest auscultation
    - Monitoring the patient for complaints of
      - pain
      - chills
      - itching
      - headache

10. What is the appropriate flow rate for an infusion of packed cells that is being run on a pump?

    40 ml/hr for the first 15 minutes, then 100 ml/hr for the remainder of the transfusion.

CHAPTER 18

1. Which component of TPN is packaged in a glass bottle?

    Lipids

2. Once the amino acids and glucose have been mixed, for how long is the solution stable?

    24 hours

3. What strength of amino acid/glucose solution can be administered either centrally or peripherally?

   3.5% amino acid and 5% glucose solution

4. Your patient is receiving PPN through a peripheral IV line. He appears to be developing an infection, so the doctor orders *Rocephin (ceftriaxone) 1 g IV q12h*. What steps will you take to carry out this order?

   Carry out the appropriate calculations to determine how much Rocephin to add to an IV minibag. (See Chapter 9.) Calculate the rate at which you will run the medications. (See Chapter 13.) Check to see if the patient has a second IV line other than the one running the TPN. If there is no second IV line, one should be started so that you can run the medication through it.

5. You will assess the access device entry point at least once per shift. What signs and symptoms will you assess for?

   Heat, pain, swelling, and redness

6. Insulin may be added to TPN solution in response to what potential problem?

   Hyperglycemia

7. What diagnostic testing is routinely carried out to monitor for the above problem?

   Blood sugar and daily glucometer

8. What potential problem can occur in patients who have compromised renal function?

   Azotemia

9. What potential problem may cause pulmonary edema?

   Fluid volume excess

10. What assessments are carried out to monitor for the above problem?

    Daily weight, strict monitoring of intake and output

Index